FROM CHANCE TO PURPOSE

An Appraisal of External Human Fertilization

FROM CHANCE TO PURPOSE

An Appraisal of External Human Fertilization

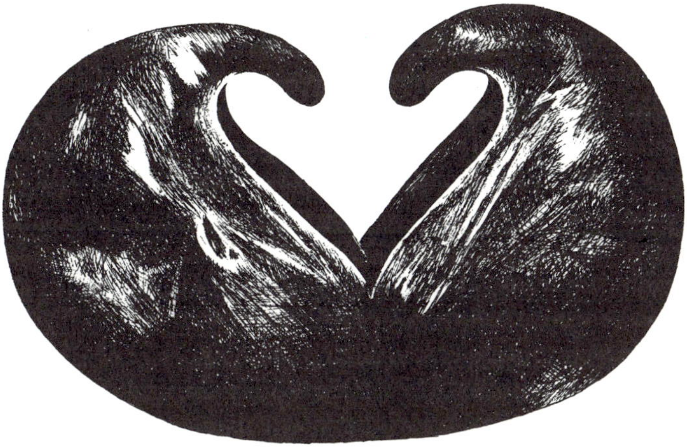

Clifford Grobstein
University of California, San Diego
La Jolla, California

1981

ADDISON-WESLEY PUBLISHING COMPANY
Advanced Book Program
Reading, Massachusetts

London · Amsterdam · Don Mills, Ontario · Sydney · Tokyo

Cover page illustration

The sculpture shown on the front cover and title page was photographed by the author during his travels. To him, it seems to convey two concepts: *twoness* reaching toward *oneness* and the sheltered and guarded space within which new life begins.

Library of Congress Cataloging in Publication Data

Grobstein, Clifford 1916–
From chance to purpose.

Includes index.
1. Fertilization in vitro, Human. 2. Fertilization in vitro, Human—Moral and religious aspects.
3. Fertilization in vitro, Human—Government policy.
4. Human biology. I. Title.
[DNLM: 1. Fertilization in vitro. WQ 205 G793f]
RG135.G76 618.1'78 81-1918
ISBN 0-201-04585-0 AACR2

Published simultaneously in Canada

Manufactured in the United States of America

I and Thou

Sine qua non

Contents

Preface

This book is about our growing capability to take life into our own hands. That growing capability raises the possibility that some day we shall be able to influence the biological nature of our own species. The possibility is not an entirely new development, nor is it immediate. However, biology and biotechnology have progressed so rapidly in this century that it is not too early to begin serious consideration of the issues raised. The next century could witness the initiation of a new epoch of human self-determination—if our civilization is not severely damaged or destroyed by the equally dramatic rise in our capability for self-immolation.

In fact, the present period may be viewed, at the dawn of the fourth millenium A.D., as the beginning of a second great human transition. The first transition was from a biological to a cultural mode of human progression. For several million years, early human life evolved by mechanisms not too different from those operating in its neighbor species. Hereditary variation occurred randomly; favorable variations persisted when they conferred reproductive advantage in particular natural environments. We call this mode of biological progression Darwinian natural selection. It is the prime mover in evolutionary change and diversification of earthly life.

The ancient strategy began to change when the human mind came to dominate the human hand—that is, when relatively simple motor activities became the implements of more complex processes such as thinking, learning, and communicating. Through these processes culture emerged—as a special, humanly created environment within which individual human lives are led. We are not the only species to create special environments that we control and that also control us and influence our subsequent evolution. Among many others, the relatively simple reef-building corals and the relatively complex colonial insects do it as well. No other environment-creating species, however, can hold a candle—qualitatively or quantitatively—to the massive environmental creations of the human species. They impact not only on ourselves but on all the organisms of the entire biosphere. Today, the evolution of virtually all life—certainly our own—is decisively affected by our self-created culture and the environmental alterations that come in its train.

Creation of artificial environments of the current scale was hardly the objective of the early humans who began the process. Nor did they give much thought to the implications the process might have for the future of the species. The evolutionary effects that have so far registered—and we are only beginning to be aware of them today—are not, therefore the products of *intention*. Rather, they are by-products of other purposes. Just as the hereditary darkening of butterflies in the English midlands was an unintended by-product of the Industrial Revolution, changes in our own gene pool resulting, for example, from medical life-saving techniques applied to genetic disease are by-products rather than deliberate creations.

However, the recent sharply rising capability for deliberate and direct intervention in hereditary and reproductive processes introduces a new dimension. Options are now on the horizon that may incorporate human purpose *directly* into human progression. In the past we made many choices without awareness or concern about hereditary and evolutionary consequences. Today certain choices are being presented for which we can no longer shift responsibility, whether to Divinity, Chance, or Unkind Fate. We are acquiring options to intervene deliberately and purposefully in fundamental matters that hitherto were beyond our control. Having long been an environment-creating species, we now face the issue of becoming a self-creating species. This is the nature of the new great transition we are approaching. We are moving from unconscious cultural determination of human biological progression to a degree of conscious self-determination.

Clearly, this second transition raises awesome issues. If human intention and purpose are to become factors in our own continuing creation, how are we to gauge their consequences? Should we be plotting long-term directions, or shall we have confidence in individual short-term decision? Should desirable directions be defined, and by whom? Are our current decision mechanisms adequate to deal effectively with the profound choices that these questions highlight? Are there principles that can be formulated to sharpen the options and guide the choices? Can the multifarious specific purposes of humanity be integrated or distilled into some consensus? Can appropriate guidelines be sustained over successive human generations? Can a "tradition" be constructed that will steer us soundly into the future when it can only be built upon past and present concurrences? Such questions emphasize that the task we face will test the highest wisdom we can muster.

The task seems to need three levels of approach. The first is primarily technical and scientific, involving the substance of the new interventive procedures and their possible futures. The second level centers on the interactions between such knowledge, decision-making institutions, and overall social purpose. The third level is the most complex of all, the question of *human* purpose itself. How can it be formulated at a time when humanity is seriously fragmented—ideologically, socially, and politically? What *are* humanity's all-encompassing aspirations with respect to its future? Can they be defined, and can they be accommodated when they are in conflict? What seems clear is that cogitation at each level must inform the other two if a total concept is to emerge.

In recognition of this necessity, the opening three chapters of this book deal first with the overall history of intervention in human heredity and development, then with the new heightened potential, and finally with the more immediate consequences to be anticipated. The fourth chapter seeks to sort the multiplicity of issues that are raised into manageable groupings for further analysis. The fifth chapter looks at a central issue of broad significance—the genesis of self and personhood. The final chapter attempts to project what we now know into future options and to deal with the requirements for sound policy mechanisms, mechanisms that may facilitate increasing consensus on purposeful choices. We cannot, at the moment, either define or write the future, least of all an ideal one. Appropriate institutional mechanisms, however, can help to assure that growing technical capability remains in continuous interaction with the most widely shared and time-tested human aspirations.

The book thus undertakes an ambitious agenda, whose full consideration will require contribution from many sources over a long period. To forestall a charge of colossal immodesty, any author seeking to deal with such issues should acknowledge the limits of his or her credentials. My professional discipline is in biology; my research career has been in the field of development. I grew up scientifically at a time when genetics and embryology had diverged widely in their areas of interest and in their methodology. However, new bridges between the two were already beginning to be built in developmental genetics and biochemical embryology. As a young scientist I became aware that the reunion of studies of heredity and development was inevitable. Accordingly, I maintained an active interest in advances in both. Today, the expected reunion has occurred, thanks to the birth and spectacular successes of molecular biology. Geneticists and embryologists alike are busy tracing the intricate interactions of nucleic acids, proteins, and other macromolecules in the transmission and expression of genetic information in both heredity and development.

These are my credentials for dealing with the scientific aspects of the subject. But what of the rest? Dare a biologist address matters of human purpose, of decision-making, and of policy formation? These are the concern of everyone and, taken together, the expertise of no one. I can only say that my activities of the past two decades have been at the interface of biomedical science and public policy. They have made me deeply aware of the vital role played by science and technology in human affairs. I have developed a special concern for the appropriate role of scientific and technical expertise in relation to public issues. I am convinced that there is need for individuals dedicated to this role—to practice what may be called science in the policy mode. Some scientists are motivated primarily or entirely to develop new understandings for their own value. Others are motivated to turn scientific understanding into technological applications. There also is need for scientists whose special function is to relate science to public issues, in no sense as final arbiter but as an essential reactant in well-informed policy-making.

This defines one objective of this book. I hope to illustrate how scientists as professional experts best fit into the process of policy-making. A first responsibility is to summarize accurately the existing state of relevant knowledge. A second is to highlight uncertainties and gaps in knowledge relating to public policy formation and, if possible and desirable, to propose ways to dispel these. A third is to examine policy options and the probable consequence of each. A fourth is to make this information available to all parties in the clearest and most useful way for each. A fifth is to present personal value judgments, if warranted, in a clearly labeled way to make sure that they do not reduce the credibility of the entire analysis for those who hold other values. To signal this, I shall use the first person singular when I recognize that I am expressing extrascientific values.

Such scientific contribution is essential to sound policy formation. Among other things, scientific evaluation can exclude imaginable options that are demonstrably contrary to verifiable fact. But it can do more. Scientific approaches can bring to common ground disputants who accept the principle of objective verifiability. In turn, this affords an opportunity to reduce conflict by following and maximizing paths of objective agreement.

These are not trivial advantages when deeply divisive ideological, philosophical, and religious values contend in a political arena. Ideology, philosophy, and religion in particular constitute deep currents in the total human outlook. They are based on long experience and tradition. The moving front of science differs from these in that it often introduces into the political arena the *latest* in human experience. Sometimes such new experiences open entirely new vistas, and often they require significant revision of outlook. This is the case with the demonstration of external human fertilization. In this instance, as in many others, science and technology are movers and shakers in relation to traditional beliefs and attitudes.

On the other hand, once accepted into a new perception of reality, the potentially common verifiability of scientific fact can bring harmony to disputes and enlarge shared outlook. This is not a claim that science can eliminate all human conflict by firmly founding every decision in objectivity alone. The human course constantly generates new uncertainties, and hence new value and judgmental conflicts, at least as rapidly as it lays old ones to rest. Humans would be less interesting and less consequential as a phenomenon in the universe if this were not so. Scientific advance contributes both to conflict-generation and to conflict-resolution. If the net conflict level is not to rise, however, special scientific attention must be directed toward assisting confict-resolution. This is the rationale for an effort to delineate a still incomplete scientific perspective on the implications of external human fertilization. Some may be concerned that to do this "in public" risks misunderstanding and unfortunate reaction. My own view is that, the sooner new realities are confronted, the sooner they will find their way into sound understanding and action.

Acknowledgments

Much that is said in this book comes from others, whether it be scientific facts or thoughts as to their significance. I have selected, ordered, and shaped the presentation, thereby also reflecting my own experience and predilection. Some sources are acknowledged in the text. If they all were, this section would be at least as long as the book—which is to say that science and its uses are very much a collective enterprise and, in the long run, largely anonymous.

Two colleagues and friends, Allen Lein and Harold J. Simon, read the entire manuscript and made valuable suggestions. My wife did likewise, as one facet of that smallest but most essential collective that is I and Thou. Arlene Winer patiently, cheerfully, and efficiently did all those things necessary to transform scribblings and drafts into a professional manuscript. Phyllis Helfand gave access to the perfect place to write a book. Barbara Hack rendered the illustrations, true in substance and spirit. Dorothea Thorburn dotted i's, crossed t's (and all the rest) to yield the polished sheen that only a skilled copy-editor can produce. Lore Henlein (publisher) made all things come together—on time. I am grateful to each of them.

Clifford Grobstein

Chapter I

Biotechnology—Taking Life into Human Hands

A birth that occurred in England on July 25, 1978, outstripped in public interest even the birth of a crown prince. The event was headlined around the world. The baby and its parents became instant celebrities. So, too, did the attending obstetrician-gynecologist, Patrick Steptoe, and his colleague, Robert G. Edwards, a reproductive physiologist. The two had collaborated for years in both the laboratory and the clinic, laying the foundation for the historic birth.

Their objective was to give new hope for children of their own to couples suffering from forms of infertility that do not prevent formation of normal eggs and sperm. What was special about the widely heralded birth was that it followed a union of sperm and egg outside the bodies of the parents without sexual intercourse.* Egg and sperm were obtained from the infertile couple and combined in a laboratory dish. In special solutions carefully incubated under controlled conditions, fertilization occurred and development began. The product of the external union subsequently was transferred to the wife's uterus. This was a medical technological feat circumventing the necessity for a natural internal process established in mammalian evolution several hundred million years ago.

It is worth recalling that nine years and five days before this unusual birth the first human footprint was set in lunar sand, an

---

*I shall refer to this process as "external human fertilization." It has also been called "*in vitro* fertilization," where the Latin version of *in glass* is a euphemism for technologically assisted. The term "test-tube babies" has also been used. With no intention to enter into terminological dispute, I choose external human fertilization as most accurately characterizing the main point—the process has been externalized, thereby rendering it more accessible and susceptible to manipulation, including intervention.

event that also stirred enormous public interest. What links the two unprecedented happenings is the rapid pace of scientific and technological advance and the premonition of novel futures that the events provide. A new array of options is opening for our species, the footprint pointing toward extraterrestrial migration, the baby toward new interventions and procedures for procreation. When these are taken together, speculative scenarios can be spun of explorations and colonization not only beyond the earth but beyond the solar system. Even without speculation, more realistic and mundane options are conceivable that are likely to stir wide debate here on earth.

There have been other startling events in recent years that have dramatized human intervention in life processes: breaking the genetic code; the Green Revolution; transplantation of human kidneys and hearts; recombinant DNA. Each may be seen individually as a bolt from the blue, without precedent, marking a new and independent initiative in humanity's powers over the natural world. But, in truth, it is the ensemble and not each individual event that is most significant. It is an important transformation in human relations with the living world. However, even this high point should not be thought to be without connections to the past. To conclude that human beings for the first time are intervening in and altering the natural course of life would be to ignore a long history and recent advances on even a broader front. This chapter seeks to set the record straight. Briefly, its message is that human "meddling" with life processes is probably as old as the human species but has in recent years reached unprecedented levels of effectiveness and power.

Meddling with Life

The recent startling events, we should also say, have not been greeted with unanimous approbation. Despite the benefits that can be foreseen from enhanced power for biological intervention, there are legitimate anxieties as well. The world of the living is sensed to be, and indeed is, very different from the physical world that we much sooner learned to mold and shape to our purposes. The living world is properly conceived as more fragile, intricate, and ephemeral than the physical. It involves forces and masses that are miniscule, although organized into dynamic functioning structures that exert major and, often, massive effects even on the physical world. But more crucial to the anxieties evoked by each new inventive thrust into life's intricacy is the fact that it is to the living world that we ourselves belong. We feel ourselves penetrated by every external impingement on vital processes; we feel the interventive knife as though it were penetrating our own person.

Therefore, the notion that life itself is becoming the target of human intervention and may become the province of a kind of engineering is an uncomfortable one for many people. Engineering arose in relation to the design and uses of large physical machines. As machines became increasingly complex, especially when they began to perform such humanlike tasks as computing, philosophical dispute was renewed as to whether living organisms are merely the most complicated of machines. The issue is better formulated as a comparison of the similarities and differences between organisms and machines. But against this background a term like "bioengineering" becomes an aggressive and even threatening presumption about the nature of life. Yet the word is increasingly heard, and for good reason.

Machines are, of course, complex tools, and tools have been from their beginning the means for more effective, purposeful human intervention in natural processes and events. Over several centuries our tools and machines have rapidly become more numerous, more diverse, and more powerful in achieving specific human purposes. Moreover, we have increasingly come to apply tools and machines not only to the physical world but to the living one—and even to ourselves. Agricultural tools that began with something as simple as the digging stick now range through combines, complex irrigation machinery, and airborne chemical sprayers. Medical tools began with the knife and herb but today include computerized whole-body x-ray scanners, laser beams, and electron microscopes. Machines are thus widely applied to intervene in and to control living processes. The term bioengineering, therefore, although it may seem presumptuous and even threatening, is a logical outgrowth of the context in which engineering began and of the expanding course it has followed.

Nonetheless, the term does carry connotations in common parlance that are excessively mechanical, out of scale, and discordant to the delicacy and subtlety of life processes. I prefer not to use it—just as I prefer not to assume that the limited similarities between organisms and machines justify the concept that human beings are usefully thought of as merely living machines. The essential point to be made does not turn on a word, however. It is an inexorable fact that, through increasing biological sophistication, we are now developing a capability to intervene in life processes that begins to approach the precision, effectiveness, and level of consequence that we associate with the most potent engineering practices in the physical world. The objectives, attitudes, and practices that underlie this interventive capability I shall refer to as biotechnology.

Biotechnology is by no means new, despite the fact that it has recently erupted over the threshold of public attention and is demanding more deliberate policy consideration. Such biotechnologies as life-support systems, pest control, and genetic and reproductive manipulation are but the recent cutting edge of the massive biological interventions that have been practiced in the past and are currently being practiced. It is important to have in mind the breadth of this spectrum of past and current practice as background for the potential hereditary and developmental interventions on humans that are the particular focus of this book.

Contemporary biology is best organized in terms of levels of organization. This concept recognizes that the living world contains wheels within wheels, to use a limited mechanical analogy. In this highly ordered world the important recognizable entities are parts of larger entities and yet themselves contain smaller ones. Individual organisms are entities within populations, populations within communities or ecosystems, and ecosystems within the worldwide biosphere. Organisms, however, also consist of subentities. These are organs that consist of tissues, tissues that consist of cells, cells that consist of organelles, and organelles that consist of molecules. To illustrate the large number and variety of human interventions in biological processes, we shall take them up in relation to entities at the several levels of biological order, beginning with the upper level—the ecosystem.

Ecosystem Meddling

Ecosystems are made up of interacting groups of reproducing populations, each population including one kind or species of organism. The populations interact directly within themselves and with each other, and they also interact indirectly through their mutual effects on a shared environment—for example, in a pond, meadow, or forest. Human intervention in such ecosystems began in the very earliest hunting and gathering stage of culture. Clearly these activities would selectively tend to alter relative numbers of species in any ecosystem whose members became a source of human sustenance. The impacts became even greater in early agricultural societies, since the simplest farming practice consists in measures to promote the rate of reproduction of a desirable species vis-à-vis less desirable ones. The effects of such interventions would be minimal overall when human numbers were small. Impacts would grow, however, as the success of agriculture allowed human numbers to increase. Growth of human populations, in turn, would necessarily lead to motivation for improved methods of intervention to obtain still higher yields of desirable organisms and their products.

This interactive process eventually led to modern technological agriculture, which is actually massive ecosystem management. The direct and intended effects are increased outputs of food and fiber relative to effort and resources expended. Involved is the deliberate creation of domesticated stocks, with advantageous characteristics for humans that often are very different from those of wild ancestral varieties. Clearing of land is also involved, thereby eliminating many natural habitats for other wild species. Fabrication of irrigation systems to increase arable land alters ground water flow and composition. These measures, combined with the extensive use of chemicals as fertilizers and pesticides, lead to a simplification of the natural ecosystem structure and to the creation of artificial ecosystems that require a continuous input of energy and materials to maintain high production levels.

Applied over large areas, these contemporary agricultural technologies have extensive effects that entirely modify, for example, the character of such vast areas as the Mississippi Basin. When combined with the results of urbanization and energized by fossil fuels, these effects can include significant changes of ambient temperature and of CO_2 concentration that are now approaching global atmospheric modification. Human interventions in ecosystems are therefore becoming significant geologic and physiographic factors, with spin-off consequences for all living species, including our own.

Thus, the most massive human intervention in biological systems occurs at the ecosystem level. No other species has ever so totally dominated the worldwide ecosphere. Efforts to counterbalance the less fortunate effects of this intervention are being made through reforestation, through preservation of wilderness areas, through special protective measures for endangered species, etc. Effective long-term husbandry rather than short-term exploitation of the ecosphere is urged as the objective of new approaches to agriculture and to management of land and other natural resources. Yet even these measures require continuing and expanding intervention to be effective. Thus, in efforts to increase the energy yield from coal to replace increasingly scarce and expensive petroleum, strip-mining of western lands threatens to cause new drastic ecological changes. Not only may denudation of forest lands result, but the diversion of water to produce transportable coal slurries may seriously compete with agricultural practices heavily dependent upon irrigation. To balance these interlocking effects will require increasingly sophisticated interventions affecting mining technology and calling for rehabilitative technologies to restore and maintain the stability of the ecosystem.

Meddling with Organisms

We intervene, of course, not only at the level of ecosystems and populations but at the level of individual plants, animals, and microorganisms as well. We have a long history—again extending back to the dim dawn of our existence—of interaction with other kinds of organisms—as food sources, as work sources, and as companions or pets. Particularly useful organisms have been domesticated—that is, incorporated into human culture. In the process, species frequently have been deliberately modified genetically, initially through casual preferential selection. Deliberate and systematic selection of desirable breeding stocks has led, over generations, not only to domesticated forms clearly different from their wild progenitors, but to sharply different types or breeds within a given domesticated kind. No one first coming upon the range of kinds of dogs—from toy poodle or pekinese to Great Dane or St. Bernard—would judge these to be all of one kind. The same can be said for varieties of cats, pigeons, horses, and goldfish. Yet all this variety within an originally much more homogeneous species results from sustained and deliberate human intervention in the breeding of these animals.

Indeed, it was this kind of breeding intervention that led to the science of genetics on the one hand, and to understanding of evolution on the other. Gregor Mendel was seeking regularities in genetic transmission of traits between generations when he undertook his classical quantitative investigations of garden peas. Charles Darwin's recognition of the correspondence between variation in nature and variation in domesticated species led to his postulate of natural selection as an equivalent diversifying factor to human artificial selection. Genetic intervention through controlled breeding, therefore, has a long history not only in relation to practical objectives but also in its contribution to scientific understanding.

Intervention in the lives of organisms is not, of course, limited to control of their breeding. Plants and animals of many kinds are the subjects of purposeful intervention in relation to nutrition, reproduction, growth, behavior, etc. In fact, there is a subclass of domesticated animals that are designated laboratory animals because they are bred specifically for investigation of their biological properties. These animals, in many instances, function as human surrogates, contributing substantially not only to our understanding of human biology but to more effective diagnosis and management of human disease. The laboratory mouse is the example par excellence. Originally developed for use in cancer research, a number of highly in-bred mouse strains—members of each strain being genetically almost equivalent to multiple identical twins—are now widely used in studies of reproduction, immunology, transplantation, and behavioral genetics.

In virtually all instances today, studies on laboratory animals precede interventions on human subjects. Resulting interventions on human beings have proceeded from simple surgical and pharmacological therapies to the elaborate procedures of modern technological medicine. These procedures now may involve multiple interventions of the most precise and probing kind. Radiation diagnosis and therapy, intravenous catheterization, brain surgery, immunization, and sophisticated life-support systems are examples of the degree to which intervention has become part and parcel of modern medical practice.

Meddling with Organs, Tissues, and Cells

Moving down another level of organization, much intervention is actually directed not at the organism as a whole but to particular organs. The heart has attracted heightened attention because of its central importance to survival. Only recently have general surgical procedures been improved to allow exposure and direct manipulation of the "open heart." Interventions on the heart are now routinely practiced, including installation of artificial pacemakers, replacement of sections of coronary arteries, insertion of mechanical valves, and transplantation of whole hearts. Efforts are even being made to replace the living heart with a truly mechanical pump.

Another example of intervention at the organ level is the blood dialysis machine, an external blood purifier serving as a substitute for a diseased kidney. Similarly, there are artificial respirators, artificial substitutes for the lens of the eye, even artificial padding to simulate the esthetic and erotic capabilities of the female breast. Endocrine products are administered in replacement therapy for diseased glands, and interventions can control reproductive capacity, whether to prevent conception or to overcome sterility. Even the brain, as already noted, is not untouched by intervention, in the form both of surgery and of psychoactive drugs.

Below the level of organs is that of tissues and cells. In the current wave of enthusiasm engendered by the newer molecular biology, the enormous progress made in cell biology in recent decades has been somewhat overshadowed. Although the universal importance of cells in all of life had been recognized before the beginning of this century, it was not until the second half of the century that a full appreciation of cell structure and function was achieved. As knowledge grew, interventions employing cells increased in number. As an example, whole blood transfusion is essentially a tissue transfer, since blood is a complex fluid in which cells of a number of kinds are suspended. Fractionation of blood into its components yields plasma and serum as fluids and platelets, red cells, and white cells as particulates. Each of these fractions and subfractions has its particular uses in intervening in human or animal disease. Blood collection, typing, processing, storage, and distribution are a major component of the health care system in every major population center in the United States.

Procedures for maintaining, growing, and manipulating cells outside the body also have been steadily improving in effectiveness. Particular kinds of cells are cultured externally in laboratory dishes and then studied for various purposes, including possible reintroduction as skin grafts or bone marrow replacements. Such exteriorized cells are also used as an aid in diagnosing cancer and in detecting genetic disease, in both instances providing a basis for other interventions that may contribute to disease control. Another cellular intervention is the use of sperm cells, frequently after storage in the frozen state, in artificial insemination leading to internal fertilization. External human fertilization is one more example of manipulation of living cells in laboratory culture. The natural union of sperm and egg cells in culture and the successful reintroduction of the developing fusion-cell into the human uterus to produce an apparently normal pregnancy is, of course, the major new intervention of great potential consequence that we shall discuss in detail.

Molecular Meddling

Finally, we come to the molecular level, where an explosion of knowledge in the past quarter-century has given detailed insight into, among other things, the structure of proteins, the nature of enzymes, and the dependence of both of these on the role of the nucleic acids as information carriers. A host of interventions has been spawned by this new knowledge. Vaccination began at an earlier period but will be made more precise and useful as new and safer vaccines are developed by molecular fragmentation and purification. Antibodies of great specificity and purity can also be produced, both for immunization and as tools for diagnosis. Antibiotics, hormones, analgesics, anesthetics, and psychotropic drugs are all interventive molecular tools extensively used in medical practice.

This quick summary of the vast array of biotechnological interventions already in effect is intended to emphasize that the genetic and developmental interventions to be discussed are not phenomena arising *de novo* but are a continuation of a long history of technological and, specifically, biotechnological intervention. Moreover, it is neither intervention *by* humans nor intervention *in* humans that is the new element. Rather, it is the potential level of effectiveness and the particular directions new interventions may take that command special attention. Especially important is the rising capability to intervene directly in the deep structure and developmental expression of life's hereditary core. When this is coupled with techniques to initiate externally the development of a new human being and with expanding capability to maintain external development of nonhuman mammalian embryos and their parts, the ensemble provides a strong platform for potential new interventive options.

We shall look more closely at this platform and some of the options in the next chapter.

GENERAL REFERENCES

Ciba Foundation Symposium 66 (New Series), Human genetics: possibilities and realities. *Excerpta Medica* (1979).

Committee on Science and Public Policy, National Academy of Sciences, *The Life Sciences.* Washington, D.C.: National Academy of Sciences (1970).

Congressional Office of Technology Assessment, *Development of Medical Technology.* Washington, D.C.: U. S. Government Printing Office (1976).

Egdahl, R. H., and Gertman, P. M., *Technology and the Quality of Health Care.* Germantown, Maryland: Aspen Systems Corporation (1978).

Fuller, W. (ed.), *The Biological Revolution: Social Good or Social Evil?* Garden City, New York: Anchor Books (1972).

Handler, P., *Biology and the Future of Man*. New York: Oxford University Press (1970).

Haring, B., *Ethics of Manipulation: Issues in Medicine, Behavior Control and Genetics*. New York: Seabury Press (1975).

Jones, A., and Bodmer, W. F., *Our Future Inheritance: Choice or Chance? A Study by a British Association Working Party*. London: Oxford University Press (1974).

Karp, L. E., *Genetic Engineering: Threat or Promise?* Chicago: Nelson-Hall (1976).

Kline, J. (ed.), *Biological Foundations of Biomedical Engineering*. Boston: Little Brown (1976).

Lappe, M., and Morison, R. (eds.), Ethical and scientific issues posed by human uses of molecular genetics. *Ann. N.Y. Acad. Sci.* **265** (1976).

National Research Council, *Assessing Biomedical Technologies: An Inquiry into the Nature of the Process*. Washington, D.C: National Academy of Sciences (1975).

Osborn, F., *The Future of Human Heredity*. New York: Weybright & Talley (1968).

President's Biomedical Research Panel, *Appendix A—The Place of Biomedical Science in Medicine and the State of the Science*. DHEW Publication No. (OS) 76-501 Washington, D.C.: Department of Health, Education and Welfare (1976).

Reiser, S. J., *Medicine and the Reign of Technology*. New York: Cambridge University Press (1978).

Chapter II

External Human Fertilization: A New Technology

The birth of a baby that is not the direct result of parental intercourse challenges and even affronts some of the deepest and most powerful traditions that underlie human behavior and society. Yet, the success of the Edwards–Steptoe procedure demonstrates that in physiological terms parental intercourse is merely a way to bring egg and sperm into the proximity necessary to undergo fusion. It is the cellular fusion that has important biological consequences, not the procedure to assure it. Such sexual fusion between cells, according to current evidence, began over a billion years ago, probably among single-celled organisms inhabiting ancient pools. The process caught on because it generated wider hereditary variation among its products, thereby enhancing the probability that some descendant cells would survive in new or changing environments. The advantages of such adaptive genetic capability became deeply ingrained and were passed on as more complex multicellular organisms evolved into the plants and animals of today. Reminiscent of that history, contemporary multicellular organisms all return to a single-celled stage to undergo sexual reproduction. The human species is no exception.

In the early multicellular organisms, and in a vast array of present-day species, natural sexual union occurred and continues to occur externally. Internal fertilization and development is a special property of mammals and some other organisms. Presumably it arose because the greater protection provided to the young reduces the number of eggs required to assure a new generation. In humans the arrangements to ensure internal fertilization have become exceedingly complex, and the period of internal development is unusually long. Beyond their biological significance, the necessary arrangements include powerful emotions, both tender and violent. They generate complex rituals and behaviors that permeate our society and have inspired an enormous literature, both sacred and profane. They are, therefore, not lightly shed when technological ingenuity circumvents them.

Persisting beneath the intricate social and psychological trappings, however, is the primordial sexual union of two cells that combines heredities and yields the unique promise of a new generation. This event is conception, fertilization, or, technically, *syngamy*. Syngamy says it best in human terms, because it stems from the Greek recognition that this is the essence of wedlock. The Greek word *syngamein* means to marry together, and appropriate modifications of the word designate a husband and a wife. The Greeks, as always, had a word for it, a word that binds together a man, a woman, and a child in what is expected to be indissoluble family union. An I and a Thou remain *sine qua non* for human genesis. Today we use the Greek word as a technical designation, but we have also created a technology that can separate totally the biological event of egg and sperm fusion from the usual preliminary behavior of the parents. Potentially we have also separated the primordial event from the emotional and social context in which it traditionally has been embedded. In this innovative technology, therefore, lies not only the potential of new constructive options but also the anxiety and resistance invariably generated by profound innovations that perturb ancient traditions.

Circumventing the Oviduct

The new technique was devised to circumvent the dependence of the processes of internal fertilization upon the oviduct. This fragile tube in the female body is the passageway both for downward transport of the egg from the ovary and for upward passage of the sperm from the vagina to the point of nuptial union (Figure 1). Any severe malfunction or malformation of the oviduct reduces or eliminates the possibility of successful internal fertilization and childbearing. Perhaps one in 500 women in the United States has an abnormality or obstruction of the oviduct that interferes with effective gametic transport (1).* Such women are sterile

*Numbers in parentheses refer to Specific References listed after the Postscript.

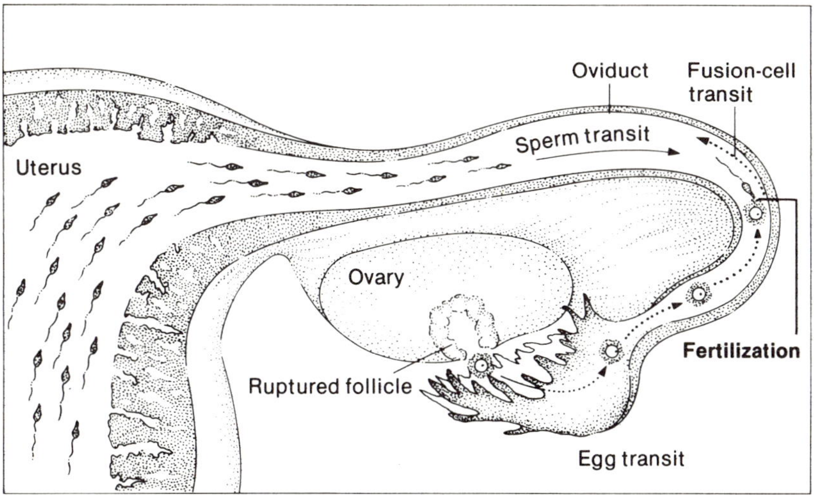

Figure 1. The oviduct as the transit track for egg and sperm to point of fertilization, followed by fusion-cell transit to the uterus. The follicle has just ruptured, and insemination has occurred some hours before. Fertilization is shown occurring, and the fusion-cell will continue down the oviduct to implant in the uterine wall.

despite the fact that they may have normal ovaries and uterus. Surgical correction has been attempted, but this required abdominal entry—to be avoided whenever possible—and very difficult and often unsuccessful repair of the fragile oviduct. Therefore, it was an attractive suggestion that the obstacle might be circumvented through less drastic surgery, by obtaining the egg before fertilization, fertilizing it externally, and then returning the fertilization product or zygote directly to the uterus.

The idea is straightforward, but realizing it is fraught with technical difficulties. It would not have appeared feasible were it not for major advances in our understanding of reproductive mechanisms derived from fundamental and practical studies on both animals and humans. Success depends on the following steps: (1) obtaining a healthy egg ready for fertilization; (2) maintaining the healthy egg outside the mother prior to fertilization; (3) obtaining healthy sperm capable of participating in fertilization under artificial conditions; (4) achieving syngamy; (5) maintaining the fertilization product outside the mother until it develops far enough to return to the uterus; (6) successful implantation of the developing egg in the uterine wall.

Understanding Human Reproduction

The accomplishment of these steps utilizes a half-century of increasing understanding of all aspects of human reproduction. Several factors have contributed to this advance of knowledge. Simple desire to know has played its role, as it does with less emotion-laden subjects. There have also been, however, a number of important practical objectives—not only in human medicine but also in animal husbandry for agricultural purposes. Achieving higher yields in production of cattle, for example, and relieving human infertility have a common knowledge base, and advances in one cross-feed to the other. Overshadowing both of these motivations, however, has been the looming impact of rapid human population growth. Among the genie popping out of the many bottles fashioned by science and technology, none has had greater impact on the future than our own enhanced capacity to increase our numbers. The need for interventions to influence the rate of human reproduction has been a major thrust of the social thinking of this century. The science of reproduction has expanded accordingly.

The thrust toward population control relies heavily on technological fixes. The frequency with which eggs and sperm meet obviously is a basic determinant of reproductive rate and population size. Biological factors—what Malthus called the passion between the sexes—act to increase the frequency of egg and sperm union. The pressure has been to understand all the events and mechanisms that contribute to the crucial meeting so as to intervene mechanically, physiologically, or biochemically to reduce the frequency—without loss of the pleasures of passion. This mechanistic assumption has provided a powerful impetus to research in reproductive biology. It has so far had moderate success in its major objective. It is a small irony that it has also spawned external human fertilization—an intervention to *increase* the chances of fertilization when natural events have reduced it.

The Reproductive Cycle

To describe the technology developed for external human fertilization, we must first outline several lines of advancing knowledge about the reproductive cycle. The first deals with the mechanisms of control of the cycle of the female mammal, and particularly of women. Involved are (Figure 2) the hypothalamus (a portion of the brain floor to which the pituitary gland is attached), the pituitary gland itself, the ovaries, the uterus, the vagina, and the breasts or mammary glands. Functions of these organs are coordinated by hormones produced by one organ and transferred to another in the circulating blood. It is increased understanding of the functions and interactions of the reproductive organs that has provided new techniques for interventions in the cycle—techniques that can increase or decrease the probability of successful meeting and union of sperm and egg.

For our purposes the ovary can be thought of as the center of the cycle, since it produces the mature egg. The egg develops from a primordial cell in the ovary that acquires a surrounding layer of accessory cells. The multicellular structure thus produced is called a primary follicle. At the onset of each cycle in humans (lasting approximately 28 days), a single primary follicle in one or the other ovary begins to enlarge, mainly by proliferation of the accessory cells. As the number of cells increases, fluid accumulates to form a cavity within the cellular mass. Enlargement of the follicle thus involves not only proliferation but accumulation of fluid. As the follicle enlarges and the enclosed egg matures, the follicle moves closer and closer to the ovarian surface. A mature follicle is like a blister at the surface, with a relatively thin wall and the egg supported by accessory cells at the outer pole of the blister. The growth and maturation of the follicle takes about two weeks, counting from the time of onset of the last menstrual bleeding.

Around the fourteenth day the follicular blister bursts (ovulation), ejecting the egg, along with a "corona" of investing follicular cells, into the funnel-like end of the oviduct or fallopian tube (Figure 1). The egg is transported down the tube by currents created by the beating of hairlike cilia on the cells lining the tube. Meanwhile, back in the ovary, the residual accessory cells of the

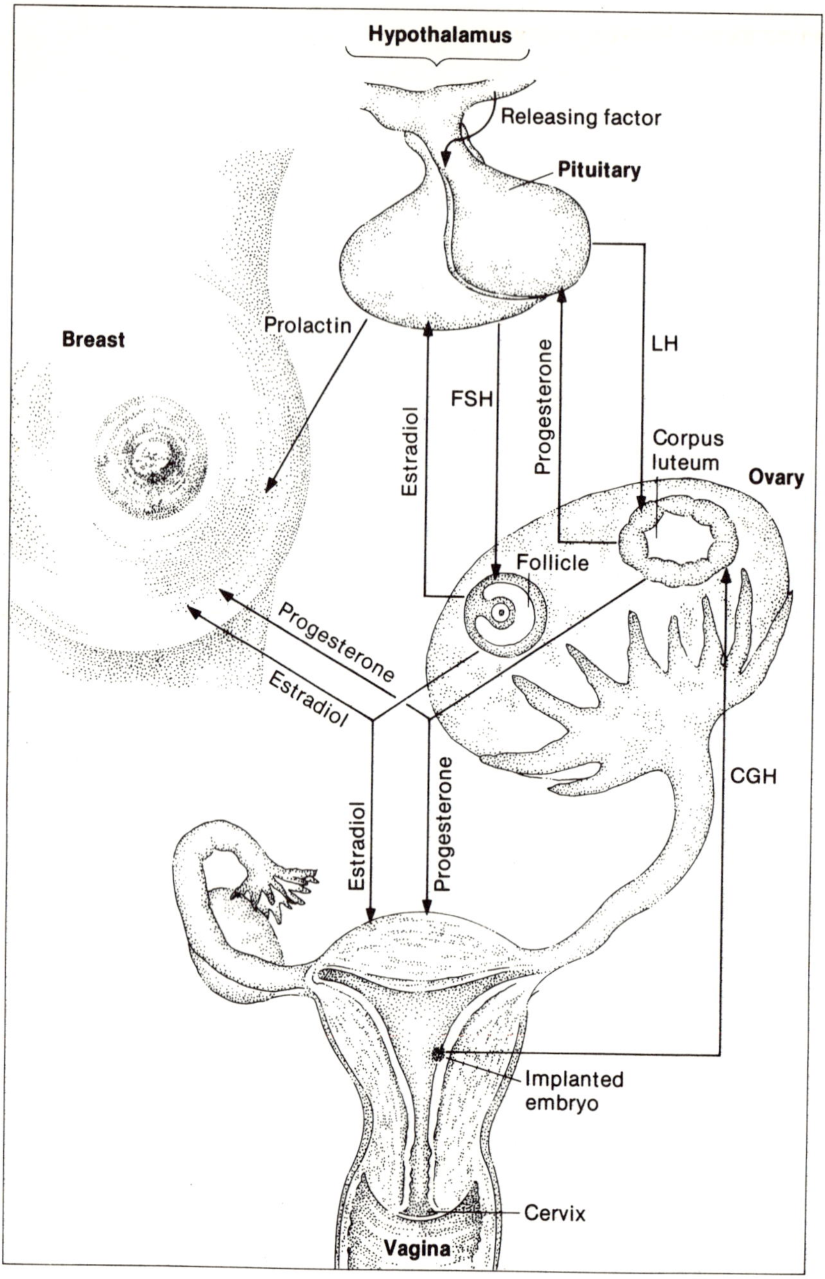
Hypothalamus
Releasing factor
Pituitary
Breast
Prolactin
LH
FSH
Estradiol
Progesterone
Corpus
luteum
Ovary
Follicle
Progesterone
Estradiol
Estradiol
Progesterone
CGH
Implanted
embryo
Cervix
Vagina

collapsed follicle are transforming in appearance and activity to form the corpus luteum (yellow body). This persists, in the absence of pregnancy, for some 10 days and then undergoes a second transformation to form the scarlike corpus albicans (white body). At the same time, menstruation begins. However, if the egg, in its transit down the oviduct, meets sperm moving upward from the vagina and uterus, fertilization may occur. The fertilized egg will then begin dividing as it moves along the oviduct and into the uterus. In this case the corpus luteum persists in the ovary for a much longer time.

These events involving the ovary allow distinction between two phases in its cycle: (1) a follicular phase up to the moment of ovulation; and (2) a luteal phase from the moment of ovulation to the beginning of menstruation or, in the event of fertilization, on into pregnancy.

Cyclic changes in the uterus are correlated in time with the events of the ovarian cycle. The outer layer of the uterine wall is muscular (the myometrium), the inner is glandular and vascular (the endometrium). At the conclusion of a menstrual period the

◀

Figure 2. Hormonal control of the reproductive cycle in female mammals. Ovarian activity is regulated by two hormones from the pituitary (FSH, LH), in turn dependent upon a releasing factor from the floor of the brain (hypothalamus). The developing follicle and the corpus luteum (formed by transformation of the discharged follicle) produce estrogens and progesterone that stimulate the uterine lining and the maturing breast. Milk production by the breast requires further stimulation by the pituitary in pregnancy (prolactin). Pregnancy also creates another hormonal source in the early embryo and the placenta. The appearance of chorionic gonadotropin (CGH) produced by the embryo is an early diagnostic sign of pregnancy and maintains activity of the corpus luteum during the first third of pregnancy.

endometrium is relatively thin and avascular. During the ovarian follicular phase endometrial cells are proliferating, vascular supply is increasing, endometrial glands are elongating and enlarging, and the entire endometrium is thickening. The changes reach maximum during the ovarian luteal phase, and toward the end of this time the endometrium is referred to as progestational (ready for pregnancy). The state includes the ability to react with a developing embryo (progestational reaction) so as to incorporate the embryo into the endometrium (implantation) and begin the formation of a placenta for maternal–embryonic exchange. If an embryo does not arrive in the uterus well before the twenty-eighth day, circulation to the thickened endometrium is markedly reduced, regressive changes begin in the glandular tissue and blood vessels, and bleeding and tissue sloughing occur. This menstrual process returns the endometrium to its relativly inactive postmenstrual state.

Hormonal Control

What mechanisms keep events in the ovary and uterus so closely coordinated? The answers lie in a complex system of chemical messengers or hormones (Figure 2). The maturing follicle, in addition to being the site of egg maturation, is a hormonal source. The accessory cells of the follicle make considerable quantities of estradiol, one of the family of sex steroids. The estradiol is discharged into the circulating blood in increasing amounts as the follicle grows. Reaching the uterus, estradiol acts on the endometrial cells to incite the characteristic proliferation, vascularization, and glandular development. After ovulation the follicular cells transform to luteal cells and shift from making only estradiol to making progesterone as well. Progesterone, also a sex steroid, stimulates the endometrium to the progestational state, including the capability to interact with an arriving embryo. Thus, through its secretion of estradiol and progesterone, the maturing and post-ovulatory ovarian follicle prepares the uterus for both implantation and nurture of a developing embryo.

The cyclic function of the ovary results, in turn, from cyclic release of hormones produced in the pituitary gland. In the absence of these pituitary hormones, no ovarian follicles will mature and, accordingly, the uterus will likewise be quiescent. One pituitary hormone (FSH) stimulates follicular growth in the ovary; a second (LH), acting after the first, induces ovulation and transformation of the follicle to the corpus luteum. Recently it has been discovered that the pituitary hormones are also subject to control, in this case by the hypothalamus, to which the pituitary is attached. The hypothalamus produces releasing hormone for FSH and LH. The releasing hormone introduces influence by the brain, through its hypothalamus, on reproductive function. Interaction of ovarian sex steroids, pituitary hormones, and hypothalamic releasing factors are essential to normal reproductive function.

Summarizing, there is a complex hormonal background that regulates egg production in the ovary and preparation of the uterus for successful internal fertilization and development. Knowledge of this background is essential to techniques for successful external fertilization and uterine implantation of the developing egg. As an example, accurate timing of the individual ovarian cycle of a candidate for external fertilization is essential if an egg is to be obtained at the optimum time for fertilization. The optimum time for fertilization is relatively short, as we know from extensive studies of the fertilization process in nonhuman mammals, other vertebrates, and even sea urchins. The fertilizability of the egg rises during its maturation in the follicle and declines subsequent to ovulation if it remains unfertilized. Eggs taken too early in their follicular maturation are either not fertilizable or are likely to respond abnormally. Over-ripe eggs also are likely to respond abnormally. The optimum time for effective normal fertilization begins just prior to ovulation and persists for only a few days thereafter.

Fishing for Eggs

In women it is difficult to recover eggs once they have been ovulated and enter the oviduct. In mice the oviducts can be flushed out surgically to obtain many fertilized eggs, as many as a dozen naturally and twice or more that number following stimulation with pituitary hormones. This procedure, however, requires entry into the abdomen and usually removal of the oviducts. It obviously is not an acceptable procedure for humans. The objective, therefore, must be to recover the egg directly from the follicle as close as possible to the ovulation time to ensure full maturity. This requires careful timing of the ovarian cycle of the subject, especially since the time of ovulation varies from person to person and even from cycle to cycle in the same person.

Timing of ovulation has also been important for contraceptive purposes, particularly in relation to the so-called "safe period" or temporary nonfertility of the female. A number of techniques have been tested in this connection, including changes in body temperature and in the character of vaginal secretions during the cycle. These are indications of the changing hormonal levels in the blood and body fluids already referred to. Techniques for detecting and measuring the hormonal changes themselves have been steadily improved in sensitivity. In particular, it is now possible, by following LH levels in urine, to forecast the imminence of ovulation within a matter of a few hours. Just prior to ovulation there is a distinct rise or "surge" in the LH urine level. When this is observed, the egg can be expected to be still in the follicle but optimally ripe for fertilization.

The ability to obtain an egg at this optimum time depends upon advances in surgical knowledge and, specifically, in gynecological techniques. Visual inspection of the abdominal organs is an important step in accurate diagnosis of a number of diseases. In the past it has necessitated laparotomy or major surgical incision through the abdominal wall. Even under modern surgical conditions, laparotomy followed by manipulative examination of the internal organs is not an inconsequential procedure, entailing significant risk and often relatively long recovery. To avoid such laparotomy the laparoscope was devised, based upon advances in fiber optics. A laparoscope is essentially a flexible bundle of quartz fibers capable of transmitting light in curved or irregular paths and of producing images by means of accessory lenses and mirrors. Only a very small incision is required to introduce its slender probe into the abdominal cavity to illuminate the contents and reflect back images to an eyepiece.

Using a laparoscope the gynecologist can examine the ovaries and locate the distinct blister of the immediately preovulatory follicle, known to be present from the earlier obtained hormonal data. A fine hollow needle, coordinated with the laparoscope, can be pushed through the follicular wall to suck the egg out. The needle can then be withdrawn and the egg deposited in a suitable solution in a laboratory container.

Incubating the Egg

Once again, advancing knowledge derived from related areas of investigation is brought to bear—in this case knowledge about how to keep various kinds of cells alive and healthy under laboratory conditions. The egg can be kept in a healthy state externally in carefully compounded solutions that are varied slightly prior to and after fertilization. The procedure for human eggs is based upon favorable results first obtained with eggs of other species. Similarly, a carrier solution for sperm was available from nonhuman studies. This solution suitably modifies or capacitates the sperm. Without this effect, normally produced by fluids in the female genital tract, the sperm are unable to participate in fertilization. Upon introduction of the capacitated sperm, the actual fusion of egg and sperm can be followed microscopically and subsequent events can be checked at intervals to detect any indication of abnormality.

Thus, a period of continuing external development under observation is critical to the procedure. Immediate return of the presumed fertilized egg to the donor would pose several potential hazards. The time, effort, and expense of reimplantation would be fruitless if the egg were not actually fertilized or were in any way abnormal. Many early attempts at external fertilization, in both animals and humans, were frustrated in this way. Moreover, there is a problem in matching reimplantation of a recently fertilized egg to the state of the recipient. Normally the developing egg would be transported through the oviduct for several days before arriving in the uterus. Return of the externally fertilized egg to the oviduct, however, is not a procedure of choice in humans because of the fragility of the duct and because it would require abdominal reentry. Implantation into the uterus via the vagina and cervix is far simpler. However, in the normal process the uterus usually is not a in a receptive state for implantation until several days after ovulation. It is not clear, therefore, that immediate return to the donor of the externally fertilized egg would provide optimal circumstances for successful implantation. Some period of continued external development of the externally fertilized egg is currently regarded as necessary both for observation and for correlating the stages of the developing embryo and the uterine cycle.

From the limited information* so far available about the Edwards–Steptoe procedure (2), it appears that the successful cases involved about two days of external maintenance and that the eggs had undergone three divisions to yield an eight-cell stage. There is some suggestion that later stages reached by longer periods of external maintenance may be less successfully implanted, but the information is still too scanty to make a useful judgment. This possibility clearly is something on which more information will be sought in the future, and it is a matter of some importance in evaluating more general implications of the procedure.

Implanting the Egg

Implantation of the developing egg into the uterus via the cervix (Figure 2) is a relatively simple step, comparable to many other procedures used by obstetrician–gynecologists and also pioneered in both experimental animals and animal husbandry. The introduced egg presumably continues development while floating for a time in the fluid of the uterine cavity and eventually makes contact with the uterine lining to initiate the implantation reaction. These events cannot be observed in humans, either in normal or in external fertilization. In both instances the earliest indication of successful implantation is provided by hormonal changes. As already noted, the corpus luteum in the ovary regresses to a corpus albicans late in the cycle if fertilization does not occur. This does not happen if a fertilized egg arrives in the uterus and implants. It is now clear that the developing egg provides the signal of its arrival in the uterus through the production in its outer layer of a hormone whose effect is similar to that of LH from the pituitary. The hormone is known as chorionic gonadotropic hormone (CGH), the chorion being the outer embryonic layer that contributes to the placenta and gonadotropic referring to a stimulatory effect on the primary sex organ or gonad, in this case the ovary. The continued production of CGH maintains an active cor-

*See Addendum, p. 149.

pus luteum in the ovary during the first third of pregnancy. Progesterone levels thereafter remain high because of production by the placenta, resulting in continuing stimulation of the endometrium and also in inhibition of the muscular contractions of the myometrium that will expell the infant at term.

Monitoring Development

The unusual circumstances of external fertilization warrant special monitoring of embryonic and fetal development to detect any deviations from a normal course. Techniques and procedures for such monitoring have been steadily expanding, and the amount and reliability of the information provided have been increasing. Included among the techniques, besides hormonal assay of blood and urine, are amniocentesis, fetoscopy, and ultrasonography. Amniocentesis involves drawing of samples of the fluids surrounding the developing embryo. It requires penetration of the abdominal and uterine wall and accurate entry into the cavity provided by the embryonic membranes. Accurate entry can be aided by ultrasonography. The fluid obtained thereby can be analyzed chemically. The fluid also contains cells derived from the embryo and its membranes. These cells can be studied microscopically, particularly to determine chromosomal composition and state as an indicator of a number of genetic disorders. The cells can also be grown under conditions of laboratory culture and subjected to sophisticated biochemical tests for normal function. These techniques are increasingly used by obstetricians and pediatricians to detect abnormalities of embryos resulting from natural fertilization. They are equally applicable for screening for possible defects in embryos produced by external fertilization.

Fetoscopy is a specialized form of laparoscopy. Like laparoscopy and amniocentesis, it is an invasive procedure requiring a probe to be inserted through the abdominal and uterine walls and on through the fetal membranes. Under these conditions it allows limited visual examination of the embryo or fetus to detect gross abnormality. Presumably it might be combined in the future with techniques for manipulating or taking tissue samples from the embryo. The technique is still in the early stages of use, and its risk level has not yet been fully assessed.

Ultrasonography depends upon imaging of ultrasound reflections. The technique is noninvasive and, unlike x-radiation, appears to have no untoward effects biologically. Like fetoscopy, it is in the early stages of application, and recent advances are providing steadily improving resolution. Although full risk assessment has yet to be accomplished, the indications are favorable that it will provide useful information at low risk levels, particularly as the embryo enlarges.

Uncertainties as to Risk

Every innovative medical procedure raises questions of risk. In almost all instances procedures are first tested on animals; indeed they usually are derived from animal studies. Animals, however, no matter how carefully chosen or extensively investigated, never provide exactly the circumstances of human clinical application. Hence the time and conditions of appropriate first use of a new clinical procedure are matters of judgment and, frequently, of debate. That is true of the new technology for external human fertilization.

In the judgment of Steptoe and Edwards, the time for clinical trial of the new technology had arrived in the late seventies. Their judgment was not casual; their views of the cautions and criteria for initiating trials had been outlined several times, and at particular length in a paper by Edwards (3) in 1974 on the moral, ethical, and legal aspects of the matter. Nonetheless, not all their medical colleagues concurred in their judgment. For example, Luigi Mastroianni, Chairman of the Obstetrics and Gynecology Department of the University of Pennsylvania, and himself an early investigator of external fertilization in humans, told the Ethics Advisory Board that "prior to proceeding [with clinical trials] in the United States, in my opinion, additional extensive studies in laboratory animals should be encouraged so that we can have a statistically valid indication of the normality of fetuses produced following uterine transfer of in vitro [externally] fertilized eggs" (4).

Mastroianni's concern focuses on the potential offspring and not on the potential mother, who, of course, is the actual subject of the procedure. This reflects the general medical consensus that the risk to the patient is minimal in comparison with that of comparable procedures and even in relation to the risk of pregnancy itself. The consensus takes into account, also, the obviously strong motivation of sterile couples to overcome almost any obstacle to have a child of their own—including considerable risk.

What of the risk to the potential offspring? The question at issue is the likelihood of significant damage to the egg, and hence to the offspring developing from it, as the result of the manipulations in obtaining the egg, the artificial conditions under which it is fertilized and undergoes early development, and the unusual manner in which it arrives in the uterus and implants. An important aspect of the question is the criterion of "significant" damage, and here, again, one faces a matter of judgment. Several circumstances must be taken into account in the judgment.

First, it is to be recalled that the natural process in humans seems to involve, and to cope with, a surprisingly high percentage of "damaged" eggs (5). Less than one-third of internally fertilized human eggs appear to reach term, most of those eliminated disappearing prior to implantation, and most of the rest being aborted shortly after implantation. Abortuses show a considerably elevated frequency of chromosomal abnormalities compared with those found in infants at term, suggesting that embryo loss screens out abnormal embryos. The screening is not complete, since infants at term show a significant frequency of various defects, among which are chromosomal abnormalities, anatomical irregularities and more subtle biochemical deficiencies. Two conclusions seem to be warranted: (1) "Damaged" embryos would not be a novelty limited to external fertilization and would not easily be distinguished from "natural" damage; (2) grosser forms of induced damage are likely to be screened out and to be recognizable only in a higher loss rate following insertion into the uterus. It is worth noting that, if there were *no* deleterious effect of the procedure, only one in three externally fertilized eggs inserted into the uterus would be expected to go to term—unless the microscopic evaluation in the external process succeeded in eliminating eggs that would be lost in the internal process.

Second, experience with nonhuman mammalian eggs in early developmental stages suggests that they are quite hardy and resistant to damage by manipulation externally—in contrast to their lower level of resistance at later developmental stages. This is true both of laboratory animals like the mouse and of agricultural animals like cattle and sheep. One cannot be sure, however, that this will be equally true of human eggs, because there are differences among species in, for example, the fertilizability and continued development of eggs under external conditions. The human egg, however, appears to be among the most tolerant of the species tested.

Third, and extremely important, are the special criteria that must be applied to the human species. In mice or cattle a heightened incidence of damage and resulting abnormality of 1% might be acceptable for intended purposes. In humans, however, even a single case is a matter of urgent concern, both ethically and legally. This is particularly true, given the inability of the damaged individual to participate in the prior decision and to give informed consent. Moreover, experience with mice or cattle can give only limited information about possible effects on peculiarly human behavioral characteristics, whether of intelligence, inner awareness, or personality.

These circumstances make for extremely difficult judgment. What seems clear is that there is not likely to be a time when available indirect information on humans or direct information on other species will be adequate to initiate external human fertilization at zero risk. The question concerns the level of risk one is willing to tolerate. On this issue there will be individual differences depending upon individual circumstances and predilections. Since those who are most risk-tolerant and motivated are already going ahead with the procedure, their experiences will gradually provide information on which somewhat better assessments of risk can be made. For more subtle effects on human behavior to be statistically validated, the time required is likely to be measured in decades.

Risk Assessment and the Open Window

There are ways to speed up risk assessment to some degree. The most cogent information necessarily comes from careful observation of human eggs, embryos, and the resulting offspring.

Observations with the optical microscope, as already conducted during research leading to the process, detect only relatively gross abnormalities. Examples of such abnormalities include entry into the egg of more than one sperm, failure of proper joining of parental chromosomes to the apparatus for cell division, and abnormality of the divisions themselves. Such information is logistically useful to avoid futile operative return of a nonviable egg to the uterus. The information is not sufficiently discriminating, however, to assure that eggs that pass the optical microscopic test may not, in fact, be less obviously abnormal although still viable on insertion into the uterus. Such eggs might come to term as abnormal or handicapped offspring.

More discriminating methods include use of the higher resolution of the electron microscope, study of so-called chromosomal banding patterns with the optical microscope, and biochemical tests for abnormal enzyme activities. These methods generally require sacrifice of the egg, however; they cannot be used on eggs that are actually to produce offspring. They would, therefore, have to be applied to eggs specifically obtained for test purposes. Moreover, ideally the eggs should be available in sufficient number to draw statistical conclusions about the effects of variations of procedure—variations intended to reduce the risk of damage to eggs that are to be actually returned to the uterus for development. In short, these would be experiments on human eggs with the intention limited to assessing risk and improving the procedure.

This is the rationale of an application for research support pending before the National Institutes of Health (NIH). The NIH found the application scientifically meritorius but, under existing regulations, was required to submit it for review to the Ethics Advisory Board of its parent organization, then the Department of Health, Education and Welfare (now the Department of Health and Human Services). The Board found the research for which support was sought "acceptable from an ethical standpoint," but its recommendation contained important caveats (see Appendix II). The Secretary of the Department still has the matter under advisement.

Whatever the Secretary decides, the issue is not likely to be finally resolved by that action alone. The matter is too complex and opinions are too conflicting for settlement by administrative fiat. What is at stake is whether human eggs should be obtained and fertilized for purposes other than the direct medical objective of returning them to the donor to relieve infertility. If they are obtained for risk assessment, they can contribute little to the alleviation of the immediate donor's problem, although they may contribute to less risk for later donors. If obtaining eggs from volunteer donors is acceptable for risk assessment of external fertilization, is it also acceptable for risk assessment in other situations? For example, there is considerable concern about the effect of toxic substances—smoking, alcohol, various drugs, pesticides, etc.—during early pregnancy. Should externally fertilized eggs obtained from volunteer donors be exposed to such substances to yield information on their risk to pregnant women and their offspring? In more general terms, should the window that has been opened on early development be used for testing that may extend widely beyond its original purpose—to overcome sterility?

These questions are immediately presented—they were dealt with very gingerly by the Ethics Advisory Board (see Appendix II). Such questions emphasize that reasonable rationales can be formulated for widening the entrée to early human development that has been created by external fertilization. It becomes important, therefore, to examine the full range of such options as they can be perceived in the light of current knowledge. A diagram (Figure 3) may help to visualize the options so far mentioned as well as those

Figure 3. Conceivable variations of human reproduction. Note that exteriorized sperm and eggs may be from either spousal or nonspousal sources. Sperm may be maintained in frozen storage in a sperm bank. Following external fertilization the period of laboratory development constitutes an "open window" for observation or intervention. The embryo may be implanted back into the original donor or a suitably "timed" nondonor. Prior to implantation it, like sperm, might be maintained in frozen storage in an embryo bank. The possibility also exists of maintaining developing embryos in culture beyond implantation stages (ectogenesis).

▶

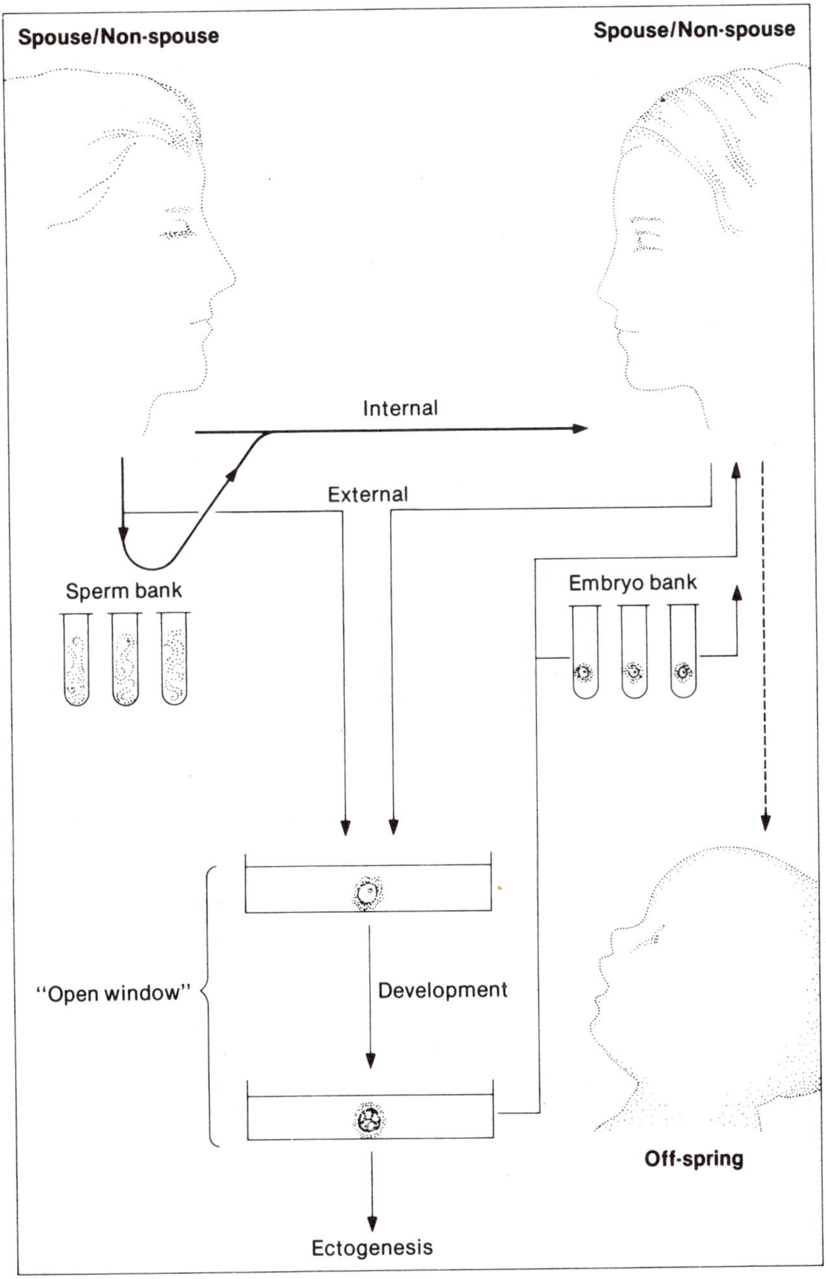
Spouse/Non-spouse
Spouse/Non-spouse
Internal
External
Sperm bank
Embryo bank
"Open window"
Development
Ectogenesis
Off-spring

that may be added. The diagram shows the basic procedure for external fertilization in relation to natural internal fertilization. It emphasizes the period between fertilization and the return of the developing egg to the uterus—the so-called open window. During this, so far, fairly short period, the embryo is accessible for observation or for various manipulations. In the next chapter we shall look particularly at the procedures applied to mouse embryos during this period, with occasional reference to other mammalian species. The studies have already made clear that there are important differences between early mammalian development and that of other animals. Human eggs, of course, would be expected to be more like those of other mammals than those of other species. The mouse therefore serves as a better human model, although not a perfect one, than the frog, the fruit fly, or the sea urchin—more traditional objects of developmental study.

Nonspousal External Fertilization

As so far reported, all instances of successful human external fertilization have involved eggs and sperm from legally married couples. Scientifically, there is no reason why the technology would be limited in applicability to spousal cases. The following variants of the basic procedure, which have been demonstrated to be successful in laboratory and farm animals, seem theoretically feasible in the human species.

Use of nonspousal sperm is an obvious possible variant, with ample precedent in artificial insemination by donor (6). A rationale for the procedure would be provided by the case of a woman with blocked oviducts whose husband was sterile because of low or abnormal sperm production. For such a couple to have a child that is at least partly their genetic offspring, external fertilization with an alternative sperm donor would be required. A related rationale would be provided by an unmarried woman with blocked oviducts who wanted her own child. There is no biological reason to doubt that, if the rationales are socially acceptable, the technology for external fertilization could be as successfully applied to nonspousal cases as to spousal ones. It is, after all, one of the defining characteristics of the human species that any two healthy members of the opposite sex can participate in a fertile sexual union.

A somewhat less simple technical variant is the converse of the use of nonspousal sperm—that is, the use of a nonspousal egg. A rationale for this would be provided by a woman whose ovaries could not produce normal eggs although her uterus either functioned normally or could be induced to normal function by hormone therapy. The technical problem would be to ensure that the recipient was in a receptive phase of her reproductive cycle at the time of implantation of an egg obtained from another woman and fertilized by her husband's sperm. This conceivably could be solved by finding a donor whose cycle was concurrent with the recipient's, a difficult task considering the other limitations on finding a suitable donor. Hormone therapy to regulate the two cycles to concurrency is another possibility, although it carries still unevaluated risks that the hormonal variations might harm the implanted embryo. Most feasible appears to be freezing of the fertilized egg or the early developing embryo to stop its development until the recipient uterus reaches its receptive stage. This is a procedure that has been used in farm and laboratory animals without any evident complications, although the circumstances and criteria of harm for animals are very different from those pertaining to human use.

To round out the variations on nonspousal external fertilization, there is the completely surrogate recipient—that is, a woman who is neither the source of the egg nor the spouse of the sperm donor. A medical rationale for the procedure would be provided by another woman whose ovaries function normally but whose uterus was removed (hysterectomy). She and her normal husband might have a child genetically their own by implanting their externally fertilized egg into a physiologically receptive surrogate "gestational" mother.

The technical problem, as in the preceding case, would be one of matching the reproductive cycles of donor and recipient. If successful, and experience with both farm and laboratory animals suggests that it could be accomplished, the procedure offers broader options. It *technically* could be accomplished whenever a pregnancy is undesirable for any reason, whether of health, esthetics, or economics. It would also provide a means for reproduction controlled entirely by genetic considerations, with egg and sperm from a selected woman and man brought together without social or emotional ties or restrictions. Such a genetically oriented procedure obviously would have broad social implications and, given sufficient time, might have significant biological consequences.

Essentially, these procedures would separate genetic parentage from gestational maternity, making possible offspring of genetic constitutions that would be unlikely or impossible under the social constraints and individual choices of natural internal fertilization. As an example, controlled inbreeding could be practiced, as with domestic animals, to emphasize particular traits judged to be desirable. This might lead to "breeds" of people comparable to those of cats and dogs. Also, by separating maternal gestational influences from genetic influences, much might be learned about the complex genesis of the peculiarly human aspects of intelligence and personality.

These last examples indicate the depth of the social, ethical, and even political issues raised by the technique for human external fertilization followed by uterine transfer, even within or only just beyond present technical capabilities. It is to be noted that the Ethics Advisory Board of the Department of Health, Education and Welfare, after careful deliberation on testimony of many expert and lay witnesses, limited its major conclusion that research involving human external fertilization and embryo reimplantation is "acceptable from an ethical standpoint" to reimplantation that involves only "gametes obtained from lawfully married couples" (Appendix II). In so doing, the Board was sidestepping some of the thornier social and ethical issues that the new reproductive technology raises.

This is not to suggest that the technology is likely soon to be used in all the variations outlined. It is important to recognize, however, that these scenarios are on the horizon, awaiting only somewhat more efficient technology and either individual or social motivation to realize them. If such motivations were coordinated, their overall effect might significantly alter directions of change in the human gene pool. If a social mechanism were devised to coordinate these motivations to fit purposes maintained over a sufficient number of reproductive generations, the biological effect might become significant. However, some measure of the likelihood and difficulty is provided by a rough estimate that something like ten generations might be required to produce clear-cut effects. This means a purposeful policy maintained over about three hundred years. The time could be shortened only by reduced generation times, a possibility that we shall later see is not entirely beyond theoretical formulation.

To summarize, the technology for external human fertilization is relatively complex and derivative from a number of lines of scientific advance. We know, at the moment, that the technology *can* be successful in producing live births. At least three cases were reported in reliable press accounts up to mid-1980.* One of them has been briefly recorded in the scientific literature (2). We do not know the frequency of successes and failures in more widespread use with regularized procedures. There is a conflict in medical opinion about the possible hazards to developing offspring resulting from the procedures used to date.

This new technology is the product of a long period of scientific advance, and future knowledge can only enhance the necessary technical capability for its use. The immediate question, then, is not whether the procedure is possible but rather to determine the circumstances, if any, under which its *use* is desirable. If there are circumstances under which it is desirable, an immediately following question is what further developments based upon it may be anticipated in the light of advancing knowledge in related areas. In the next chapter we shall begin to examine possible further options for intervention in human heredity and development, assuming the "open window" on early human development provided by external human fertilization. We shall approach this by reviewing what we are currently learning about mammalian development, particularly in the mouse.

*See Addendum, p. 149.

GENERAL REFERENCES

Betteridge, K. J. (ed.), *Embryo Transfer in Farm Animals.* Monograph 16, Canada Department of Agriculture, Ottawa, Ontario (1977).

Daniel, J. C. Jr. (ed.), *Methods in Mammalian Reproduction.* San Francisco: Freeman (1978).

Ethics Advisory Board, *HEW Support of Research Involving Human in Vitro Fertilization and Embryo Transfer, Appendix.* Washington, D.C.: U.S. Government Printing Office (May 4, 1979). (Referred to in this volume as EAB-Append.)

Graham, C. F., The production of parthenogenetic mammalian embryos and their use in biological research. *Biol. Rev.* **49**: 399–422 (1974).

Grobstein, C., External human fertilization. *Sci. Amer.* **240**: 57–67 (1979).

Gwatkin, R. B. L., *Fertilization Mechanisms in Man and Animals.* New York: Plenum (1977).

Lein, A., *The Cycling Female.* San Francisco: Freeman (1979).

Chapter III

Views through a New Window

The successful clinical technique for external human fertilization, as we saw in the last chapter, has opened a window on early human development. In the past, human preimplantation stages became available for observation only through an unusual combination of circumstances for gynecological surgery. Professor John D. Biggers of Harvard University pointed out to the Ethics Advisory Board in 1979 (7) that our information about human preimplantation eggs and embryos came from only fifteen specimens recorded in the world literature. Reluctance to invade or intrude upon the human body, unless required to give relief to an afflicted patient, justifiably kept the early human embryo cloistered in a very rarely opened "black box."

External human fertilization, however, appears to be on the verge of becoming an accepted medical procedure. It offers a distinct benefit to an afflicted patient under the patient's fully informed consent. As noted in Chapter II, the procedure requires recovery of a healthy, mature egg from the ovary and its fertilization externally, followed by observation of external development for two or more days. This period of observation is necessary to exclude gross abnormality and to time properly the insertion of the developing egg into the uterus. These medical requirements, if they are socially acceptable, will for the first time frequently open a window on early stages of human development. If the process is widely used, we can expect, at the very least, a considerable increase in clinical familiarity with these early stages. What options beyond this will be provided is a matter that will be decided by the directions of technical advance, by continued assessment, and by appropriate policy decision.

This chapter will discuss the range of options that may be reasonably anticipated to develop in the future. It will review what is currently being studied and discovered about the early development of the mouse, the mammalian species most widely used for developmental studies. The knowledge being gained about this small laboratory animal certainly will contribute importantly to our understanding of human development. The question is whether these new insights will generate new options for beneficial interventions in human development, options that may be so attractive that they cannot be disregarded. The discussion of options will be in the spirit of anticipatory assessment, to inform about, but not to prejudge, the many serious, nonscientific issues that will be considered in later chapters.

Mouse Development to Implantation

We begin by outlining the major steps in early mouse development, steps that are similar to but not identical with those in the human. The reproductive cycle of the mouse is short, four to five days. There is no menstrual period. The female is "in heat" on only one of the four or five days, meaning that she will accept insemination by a male only on that day, close to the time when ovulation occurs. Ovulation occurs in both ovaries, yielding a half-dozen to more than a dozen mature eggs. The number of eggs can be doubled by pretreatment with gonadotropic hormones. If insemination has occurred, the eggs are fertilized near the top of the oviduct and begin development as they move down toward the uterus (Figure 4). As in humans, the transit time in the oviducts is several days, during which the fertilized egg undergoes divisions without intervening growth periods—the process known as cleavage. Thus, eggs at one, two, four, eight, and later stages can be flushed out of the oviducts by surgical procedures at increasing times after fertilization. Much of the observation and experimentation to be described utilizes such eggs, carefully incubated in special appropriate solutions, and often inserted into the uterus of other mice to complete development.

Cleavage eventually leads to a ball (morula) of a hundred or more cells within the original egg envelope. The ball begins to enlarge when fluid, secreted by the cells, makes its appearance in the interior. At about this time the egg "hatches"—that is, divests itself

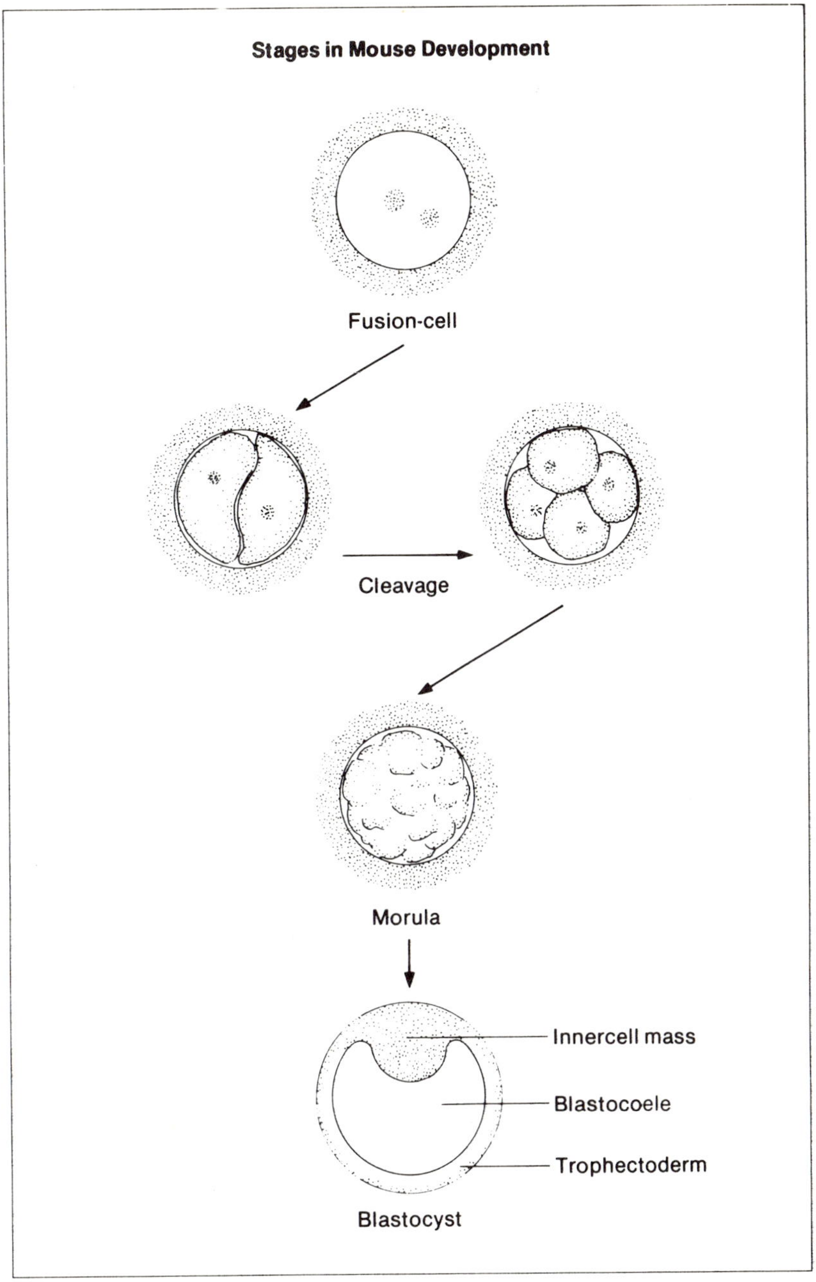

Figure 4. Preimplantation stages of mouse development. Implantation normally occurs at the blastocyst stage.

of its surrounding membrane. Accumulation of fluid soon hollows the ball, yielding a peripheral cellular wall surrounding a fluid-filled chamber. At one pole the cellular wall is thickened, projecting a knob of cells into the cavity. At this stage the young embryo is referred to as a *blastocyst*, its outer wall being the *trophectoderm* or feeding layer, the polar knob the *inner cell mass*, and the cavity the *blastocele*. Embryos are at about this stage when they arrive in the uterus. When they contact the uterine wall, they evoke a reaction that allows the blastocyst to penetrate into or embed within the wall in close association with blood vessels and endometrial glands. At this point some of the peripheral trophoblast cells of the blastocyst enlarge and migrate into the maternal tissue, expanding the area of interaction and leading toward the formation of the placenta—the specialized exchange organ between embryo and mother. At the time of implantation, too, a hormonal signal goes to the ovary to maintain the corpus luteum and its hormonal output. Pregnancy is now well established.

Using relatively low-power microscopy, special micromanipulators, and a number of biochemical techniques, mammalian embryologists have been getting information on various aspects of preimplantation mouse development. We shall focus here mainly on matters that are pertinent to human development and especially on procedures that might be coupled with external human fertilization or are relevant to the issues that it raises.

Becoming One Mouse

The first matter has to do with the time of origin of singleness, as a factor in the important concept of individuality. The fertilized egg is, of course, a single cell. It is, however, a fusion-cell derived from egg and sperm of two parents. In both mouse and human life history the single fusion-cell is unusual in being the antecedent or progenitor for all cells of the complex, multicellular adult. When the fusion-cell divides to produce two cells (blastomeres) half its size, each might be limited to forming only half an embryo. Alternatively, the cleavage could produce two equivalent cells, each able to produce a smaller but whole embryo. A similar possibility exists at the second and third cleavages. At the eight-cell stage, if all three cleavages produce like products rather than dissimilar ones, each of the eight cells would have the same capability in continued development. On the other hand, if each cleavage produced dissimilar products, each of the resulting eight cells might have its own distinctive capability for further development. Each might, perhaps, produce only one-eighth of the resulting adult.

To distinguish between these two alternatives, advantage is taken of the fact that, prior to the eight-cell stage, the cells can be readily separated and recombined with each other by means of biochemical treatments and microsurgery. One can delete one cell from a four-cell stage, add one of the four cells to another four-cell stage, or even fuse two entire four-cell stages to make an eight-cell embryo. None of these procedures changes the ability of the resulting aggregate to produce a *single* normal embryo. Moreover, addition of a cell from a four-cell stage to a later-stage blastocyst does not interfere with production of a single normal embryo.

These results would not be expected if any of the first several cleavages were unequal—that is, if they produced cells of differing developmental capability. The conclusion drawn is that the singleness or individuality of the fertilized egg is that of a cell and that its first several divisions yield products that are similarly cells, each able to give rise to any part of the adult individual. Correspondingly, an intact four-cell stage is not yet fixed to the subsequent production of a whole individual, since if two embryos of this stage are fused they jointly give rise to a single whole—in the process each producing only half of what they otherwise would have produced. The logical conclusion is that during the early stages of cleavage the oneness or wholeness characteristic of an adult mouse has not yet appeared. There is evidence, in fact, that even at the blastocyst stage the inner cell mass can split to form two embryos (8), and inner cell masses of two blastocysts can be combined to yield a single embryo. We shall return to this matter later in relation to the time of appearance of individuality in human development.

The second point to be made about mouse development elaborates on the first. There are substantial reasons for regarding the eight-cell stage as marking a significant change in the developmental status of the embryo. Prior to this stage, individual cells tend to be spherical and to show little sign of mutual adhesiveness. At the eight-cell stage a phenomenon known as compaction occurs. It is characterized by shape-changes of the cells toward a more columnar form, in turn permitting a tighter fitting-together. At the same time the electron microscope shows the appearance of so-called intercellular junctions—specializations of the surface membranes of apposed cells known to be associated with both physical adhesion and intercellular exchange of substances.

These new features of the eight-cell stage fit the idea that before this process occurs the cleavage cells are a loose aggregate of individual cells rather than a cohesive whole. Multicellular integrity begins to be acquired during the eight-cell stage.

Yet even then it is not complete, since, as noted above, an inner cell mass—which gives rise to all of the embryo at a later time—can be combined with another to produce a single individual. Moreover, identical twinning, which occurs at regular but low frequency in humans and normally produces quadruplets in the armadillo, is believed to involve splitting of a simple inner cell mass to produce multiple individuals. Clearly, there is no fixed multicellular individual yet established in the blastocyst stage. This means that suitable interventions can produce artificial identical twinning in mice and conceivably in humans. It should be noted, parenthetically, that multiple *nonidentical* births have been produced in humans—through natural internal fertilization—by hormonal intervention to overcome sterility.

Tracing What Gives Rise to What

Transfer of blastomeres from one embryo to another and fusion of two embryos to form one are now standard experimental techniques in studying early mouse development. The techniques may be used to follow the developmental fate of individual cells or to determine the interaction among cells in determining adult properties. This is done by making combinations between embryos from different strains having different genetic "markers." For example, four-cell embryos from strains having two different fur colors may be combined and inserted into a recipient uterus.

The result is an adult mouse with fur patches of each color. This result makes it clear that pigment cells of the mosaic skin have descended from one or more of the blastomeres of each four-cell stage and that the genetic traits for coat color are faithfully expressed by each cell independently of those of its neighbors. Of interest is the fact that cells of the two types are not evenly dispersed in the skin but occur in patches predominantly of one color. This suggests that, although the descendants of at least two blastomeres contribute to skin, at some point descendants of an individual cell remain together to produce a patch. Variations of the experiment, particularly those using available markers other than pigment, can give information about the time and place of origin of the specialized cell populations that make up the various tissues and organs. In turn, this pinpoints where we should look to study the mechanisms of specialization or differentiation of cell populations.

In one case (9) these methods were used to determine how many blastomeres contribute to the cell population that makes up the embryo proper, in distinction to the placenta and the extraembryonic membranes. The principle is statistical, based on the fact that not all offspring produced by fusing two four-cell embryos show mosaic coat color. If all eight blastomeres give descendants to the embryo (and hence to the skin), all offspring should be patchy; if only one gives descendants to the skin, none should be patchy, and half should be one color and half the other. In fact, patchiness and unicolor offspring of each color occur in particular frequencies, suggesting that more than one but fewer than eight blastomeres contribute to the embryo.

By extending the analysis to combinations of three and even four strains, each with different markers, one can obtain an accurate estimate of the number of blastomeres in cleavage stages whose descendants contribute to the skin or to any other tissues or organs. It is worth noting, incidentally, that in making these combinations one is producing mouse offspring that in a sense have more than two parents. Since each four-cell stage has two parents, when one fuses embryos of four strains (as has been done in a few cases), the resulting offspring contains cells genetically derived from eight parents. This is not, of course, the same meaning of parent as the ordinary one in which a genetic contribution is made to *each cell* of the offspring. But if, for some good reason, the technique were to be applied to human eggs and the resulting offspring were raised, tracing familial relationships would be complex—particularly since the ovary and testis may also be mosaic, adding to the genetic variety of eggs and sperm produced.

A possible rationale for at least limited application of cell transfer between early human embryos is suggested by another experiment carried out on mice (10). As in all species studied, there are mouse mutations that produce viable hereditary changes in single dose (heterozygous) but are lethal in individuals having a double dose (homozygous). The first such mutant identified in the mouse, called the yellow mutant, produces a yellow coat color in heterozygotes but terminates the life of homozygotes by the fifth day of pregnancy. The site and mode of action of the mutant yellow gene are not known, and there is considerable theoretical as well as practical interest in learning more about it, particularly given the high rate of loss of early human embryos referred to earlier. To test for the site of action of the mutant gene, inner cell masses of embryos resulting from a cross of two yellow heterozygotes were individually transferred into the blastocyst cavity of normal embryos.

Under such circumstances, one-quarter of the implanted inner cell masses would be expected to be homozygous and might undergo early death. In fact, their viable cells could be detected by suitable markers in chimeras at developmental times far beyond that of the death of whole homozygous yellow embryos. It therefore seems that the lethal defect is not in the cells of the transferred inner cell mass that gives rise to the embryo itself. The alternative is that the lethal gene is expressed in the trophectoderm, as was, in fact, suggested by earlier data. Death of the trophectoderm would, of course, interfere in essential interactions between the implanted embryo and the maternal tissue, leading in turn to secondary death of the inner cell mass.

Further study should now be focused on the trophectoderm to learn more about how the yellow gene exerts its lethal effect. The method also could be applied to similar genetic phenomena in the human species, either indirectly or directly. For example, although the logistics would be difficult, cells of human spontaneous abortuses might be tested for viability and developmental capability by implantation into mouse blastocysts. Such interspecific transfers have been made and have undergone limited continued development.

Transfer of Teratocarcinoma Cells

That this use of mouse blastocysts has important potential is illustrated by another line of investigation involving mouse teratocarcinomas. Teratocarcinomas are a special kind of cancer that were first studied experimentally in the testes of certain strains of mice but now can be induced in other strains in several ways. They appear to arise from early embryonic cells, the common precursors to various tissues of the body. Conforming to such origin, teratocarcinomas give rise to jumbled masses of otherwise normal cell and tissue types. The jumbled differentiated masses are nonmalignant in themselves and are referred to as teratomas. In addition, however, teratocarcinomas have a persistent complement of germinal cells that do not become specialized but continue to proliferate. It is this component that makes the tumor malignant and continuously propagable.

When grown in culture or injected as a cell suspension into the abdominal cavity of mice, the germinal cells overgrow the other types and can form a continuously propagable strain of purely germinal cells. Depending upon the conditions to which they are exposed, these cells may remain germinal or undergo specialization, making them extremely useful as subjects of studies on the mechanisms of cell specialization. When they remain germinal, however, under appropriate conditions some strains do something else of great interest. They collect into small multicellular aggregates that resemble blastocysts. Their outer wall takes on some characteristics of primitive endoderm (precursor of embryonic membranes), and the interior cells appear to become primitive ectoderm (precursor to the embryo proper). On implantation back into a mouse, these so-called embryoid bodies become typical teratocarcinomas. If, however, germinal cells or embryoid bodies are inserted into the cavity of a normal blastocyst and the combination is implanted into a uterus, the teratocarcinoma cells may be incorporated into the developing embryo and behave as normal cells. In the process they can introduce new genetic information into the embryo; in a few instances, this information has been reported to be present in germ cells and to be transferred to a succeeding generation.

This set of behaviors makes an understanding of mouse teratocarcinomas very important in relation to both normal and malignant developmental processes. It also raises the possibility of their use as vectors for genetic transformation. The apparent reversion to normalcy when cell specialization occurs recalls the well-known fact that most highly malignant tumors are without the specialized characteristics of their tissue of origin. Reversal to normalcy is not, however charcteristic of tumors in general. The relation between malignancy and cell specialization clearly needs to be better understood. Studies leading to this understanding should be carried out largely on mouse or other animal embryos. But sooner or later questions may arise in relation to human clinical problems that can most cogently be addressed by using human cells. Accordingly, human teratocarcinomas are now receiving heightened attention. Are their properties similar to the remarkable ones of the mouse teratocarcinomas? Since there are necessary and proper limits to human experimentation, can human teratocarcinoma cells, carried in culture (or in so-called nude mice that will tolerate foreign cells), be tested for reversion to normalcy in mouse blastocysts? Can this question ultimately be tested in human blastocysts? Can and should carefully controlled intervention in human blastocysts assist us to a better understanding and control of human cancer? Although there are obvious caveats, there are equally obvious rationales for carefully considering such questions.

Ectogenesis—Partial and Complete

The preceding discussion has implicitly raised the subject of ectogenesis. The term was coined to designate external development, more specifically that of human beings. The concept has been used in Orwellian terms, implying full external development of human infants in "test tubes." It is used here in the more general sense of external development, in whole or in part, of any whole organism or its parts whose development is normally internal. In this sense the Orwellian concept is one of complete human ectogenesis.

Ectogenesis may be less than complete, however, and in two ways. Development of a whole individual may be maintained externally for only part of its normal course. In that sense partial human ectogenesis has already been demonstrated for the first several days and approximately the last several months of development. The first several days have been achieved in the Edwards-Steptoe procedure, and the last several months are the achievements of intensive-care nurseries in maintaining viability of prematurely delivered infants. The other meaning of partial ectogenesis refers to developing organs or other parts of embryos maintained externally during periods when the development would normally be internal. This achievement is the product of what is called organ culture, in distinction to cell or tissue culture. It involves arrangements to externalize developing rudiments in early stages so that they can be more conveniently observed, manipulated, and analyzed as they form and mature.

Ectogenesis of whole mouse embryos has been carried successfully from the two-cell to the early somite stage. This means that mouse embryos have developed externally beyond the blastocyst stage when they would normally implant. They have continued on through the complex process of axiation—that is, the establishment of the main body axis and the major rudiments associated with it. The somites are cell aggregates that appear successively from head to tail on either side of the forming central nervous system. They later give rise, among other things, to the backbone. As the somites begin to form, the swelling of the early brain can be recognized ahead of them, and the heart rudiment is beating below. This is a stage when the primary organization of the embryo has been completed and the organogenesis that fills in the body structure in detail has begun.

This achievement was reported in 1974, but the results were inconsistent. By 1979 (11), improvements in methods allowed about 60% of single blastocysts in individual culture dishes to reach this stage in eight days of culture. Among the required components of the nutrient medium for this effectiveness is blood serum obtained from human umbilical cords, the natural circulating medium of human embryos. For reasons that are not clear, serum from other species does not work as well. It is also not clear how far beyond this point refinements of technique can extend external mouse development. With a different technique, however, rat embryos of a little earlier stage, just prior to somite formation, have been reported to progress to the 26-somite stage in 48 hours (12). This is a significant advance because the stages covered are a critical period for the main processes of organogenesis. Even if whole embryos cannot develop further than this without establishing something equivalent to a placental circulation, organ rudiments obtained from the whole embryos might be carried to greater maturity in an organ-type culture.

In fact, a number of early organ rudiments of the mouse have been sucessfully cultured from their earliest appearance to a reasonably mature state. This kind of partial ectogenesis of the mouse and other mammals is well established as a technique for analyzing interactions among organ components, specialization of cells, hormonal effects, mechanisms of tumor formation, specificities of neural connections, and toxicity of various synthetic materials. Although complete ectogenesis of any species is at least some distance away, partial ectogenesis is well along. If various fragmentary procedures that have been individually reported can be successfully combined in one species, reasonably mature organs might soon be produced externally—albeit in several steps—from a fertilized egg. Among the organs that are being extensively investigated and might be included is the ovary. Successful external maturation of the ovary and its follicles could provide a supply of eggs for external fertilization without surgical intervention.

Frozen Storage of Embryos

Ectogenesis can widen the window of accessibility to mammalian developmental stages in general. The freezing and storing of embryos also can contribute to accessibility and manipulability. For example, frozen embryos of farm animals can be transported around the world far more cheaply than can the adult animals, allowing new strains to be more easily introduced into wide use. It has been noted, also, that matching of the developmental stage of the embryo to the physiological state of the recipient uterus is a matter of concern in external human fertilization. If the embryo develops more slowly externally, or if gonadotropic hormones used to support or increase ovulation temporarily alter endocrine balance in ways that might adversely affect the implantation process or the implanted embryo, there might be some advantage in postponing implantation of the embryo until a later cycle.

Freezing of living cells, tissues, organs, or, conceivably, whole organisms is the subject of cryobiology, widely investigated in the past decade or two. Although there is much yet to be learned, particularly about species differences, it is clear that freezing need not terminate life but can essentially suspend it. Requirements for success include the nature of the suspending medium, the rate of freezing, and the rate of thawing. A major advance was made with the discovery that adding glycerol to the medium gives considerable protection to cells and tissues. Another major advance was the realization that formation of ice crystals is damaging to cells and tissues. With these precautions, cells and tissues of a number of species can be stored in liquid nitrogen at −196°C. Such cells and tissues, on appropriate thawing, show neither alteration nor damage.

These techniques have been applied successfully to embryos of a limited number of farm and laboratory animals, including the mouse. For the mouse, the procedure is advocated as a means of economical storage of a wide variety of experimentally valuable mutants and strains that have been accumulated over the years. Without such storage, animals must be continuously bred to maintain these mutants and strains. A number of individual laboratories have already resorted to freezing of embryos to reduce space and labor needs. Central embryo banking would further reduce costs and assure wider accessibility. Similar practices would offer comparable advantages for commercially valuable embryos. Studies on mice (13) suggest that storage for 200 to 1000 years would be required before minimal deleterious effects might be expected due to background radiation at current levels. Genetic changes due to radiation are the only ones to be expected at such low storage temperatures. The technique should therefore be applicable to preservation of valuable genetic stocks of all kinds, including endangered species. Although as yet there are no reports that this technique has been attempted with human embryos, on the basis of experience with animals it seems likely that it could be successfully applied.

Nuclear Manipulations

For a century or more, the cell nucleus has been understood to be of special significance in heredity and development. Understanding came originally from microscopic observations on nuclear behavior—in dividing cells, in the formation of sperm and eggs, and in various "natural experiments" in life forms that display unusual nuclear behavior. In the past several decades, microsurgical and other procedures have been elaborated that allow nuclei to be directly manipulated and to be excised from or implanted into living cells. In the last decade these interventive procedures have begun to be used on mammalian eggs.

Normal development cannot proceed very long in the absence of a nucleus. Given the fact that the nucleus is the site of most of the cell's DNA and, therefore, of its genetic information, the essentiality of the nucleus for continued development is not surprising. Nor is it surprising that in sexual reproduction an early step is the production of a fusion-nucleus derived from both parents. More noteworthy is the fact that development does not require a fusion-nucleus but can be supported by the egg's nucleus alone. This was first recognized in a "natural experiment," in species in which eggs normally develop without fertilization—that is, parthenogenetically. In some insects and in a number of other invertebrates parthenogenesis is a regular feature of the life cycle. In vertebrates it is far less common and so far as is known, with the possible exception of the turkey, does not ever lead to normal offspring. But a number of nuclear manipulations, including the equivalent of parthenogenesis, have recently been carried out on mouse embryos to yield unusual offspring.

Parthenogenesis does occur naturally in a small percentage of eggs in the mouse ovary, with subsequent cleavages but terminating in early death. In one strain of mice, called LT, this occurs with unusual frequency, and the eggs often implant before dying. There also is reason to believe that teratocarcinomas, occurring in both the testis and the ovary, may involve parthenogenesis-like nuclear changes. Recently, nuclear transfers between mouse eggs have shown that actual uniparental development can be produced by combined microsurgical and biochemical procedures (14).

There are two requirements for the initiation of development in the mouse. The first is activation of the egg to break the state of arrest that exists on completion of maturation of the egg in the ovary. This normally occurs on entry of the sperm. The second requirement is to restore the diploid chromosomal state. Both egg and sperm are in the haploid state with 20 chromosomes, each chromosome having a fraction of the total nuclear genetic information necessary for development. The diploid state has 40 chromosomes, made up of 20 homologous pairs that provide a double complement of the necessary genetic information. Diploidization is normally accomplished when the haploid complements provided by the egg and sperm of the two parents are combined in the fusion-nucleus.

Both requirements have recently been met in uniparental reproduction in the mouse in the following way. Newly fertilized eggs were obtained either by flushing them out of the oviduct after natural internal fertilization or by external fertilization. In either case, the egg already had been activated by entry of the sperm. Under the optical microscope, two so-called pronuclei can be observed, one being the egg nucleus, the other the product of expansion of the newly introduced sperm head. Each pronucleus contains a haploid set of chromosomes. One pronucleus can be removed with a micromanipulator. By treatment of the egg with a substance that alters the behavior of the division apparatus, division of the cell can be postponed until after each of the pronuclear chromosomes has duplicated—that is, until the 20 chromosomes have doubled to produce 40. With the diploid chromosome state thus restored, the egg can then be allowed to cleave normally to form a diploid embryo whose chromosomes are derived from only one parent.

The procedure has two consequences for the resulting viable embryo. First, it can only be female because it will have two identical sex chromosomes—the so-called XX constitution that determines femaleness in mammals. One can be sure of this, because if a Y-bearing sperm pronucleus had remained in the egg, the embryo would be YY, a nonviable chromosomal constitution in the mouse. Second, the embryo would have to be homozygous—all of its chromosome pairs would be identical, since they would be replicas of the 20 received from the female parent. In turn, this would mean that any genetic defects carried in from the mother would be present in double dose and would be expressed in the offspring. In the highly inbred mouse strains used in the experiments so far, the number of such genetic defects would be expected to be low. In non-inbred organisms—for example, humans, where the average number of lethal defects is estimated to be about five—the number of viable embryos would be sharply reduced.

Such embryos as might survive, however, would be immediately equivalent to or beyond the highest degree of homozygosity obtainable by inbreeding after about twenty-five generations of brother-sister mating. The high degree of homozygosity would mean that, if the resulting offspring were fertile and their eggs were subjected to the same aborted fertilization, all descendants would be genetically identical—that is, clones. Descendants would remain genetically identical, if reproduced in the same way, except for effects of mutation. Among other special properties, such mice would all be universal donors among themselves for blood and all other cells, tissues, and organs.

The production of human clones has, for some reason, caught the fancy of many people, including the press. Interest began when artificial cloning was accomplished in a different way from that just described. Frogs and toads have much larger eggs than mammals; they are, therefore, much more readily manipulated. Accordingly, they have been a favorite experimental material for developmental study. Some years ago the question arose whether the differentiation of cells that occurred following cleavage was due to parceling out of nuclear genetic factors during cleavage. If so, later-stage nuclei should be different from each other and from the fusion-nucleus that gave rise to them. To test this, the fusion-nucleus was removed after fertilization, and nuclei from later stage cells were inserted in its place. The result was clear-cut for nuclei through and beyond cleavage—these nuclei had not lost their ability to produce descendants for all of development, and nothing had been parceled out irretrievably in the cleavage process. Concerning full stages of later differentiation, controversy persisted. What was clear, however, was that the process of nuclear transplantation from a single multicelled donor could be used to introduce identical genetic constitutions into a number of eggs. Such eggs should produce the equivalent of identical twins—that is, a clone.

Several years ago a book appeared purporting to record the success of such a procedure in humans (15). Professional biologists scoff at this claim. Nonetheless, technical steps have recently been recorded in the mouse (16) that move part way toward achievement of mammalian cloning on the model of the frog. A nucleus from a mouse blastocyst cell was transferred into a fertilized mouse egg, and then *both* pronuclei were removed. The egg cleaved to produce a blastocyst that was inserted into the uterus of a recipient female mouse. By this procedure three offspring have been born with a genetic marker corresponding to the donated nuclei. The procedure could yield clones if multiple nuclei from the same blastocyst were inserted into a series of eggs.

It is not clear, however, that nuclei from an adult would work in the same way as blastocyst nuclei. In fact, trophectoderm nuclei do not work, suggesting that this earliest differentiation alters the nucleus. Success in later stages may very much depend on which cells are selected as donors of nuclei. Nuclei from human spermatocytes (diploid cells prior to production of sperm) have been recorded, although without convincing validation, to have been transferred to human eggs that subsequently underwent cleavage (17). Certainly nuclei from this source would be expected to have the highest probability of functioning in successful cloning. It can be anticipated that nuclei from such sources in mice will be tested in the not-too-distant future, since this approach should yield information on the still disputed question of nuclear change in relation to differentiation mechanisms. As an example, the technique has already been used to test the normalcy of the nuclei of LT mice that undergo partial development parthenogenetically. Such nuclei, transferred to fertilized eggs of another mouse strain, are able to participate in normal development. The failure of LT parthenogenetic eggs to continue development (14) is not, therefore, the result of a nuclear defect; a parthenogenetically produced nucleus can function fully in a normally fertilized egg.

Recombinant DNA and Genetic Intervention

The window opened by human external fertilization may afford at least one other opportunity for intervention in human heredity and development. This opportunity has recently been reported in press accounts to have been validated on mouse eggs. It was earlier foreshadowed in experiments on adult mice. To understand the rationale, we must briefly review the procedures that are referred to as recombinant DNA technology.

DNA is the fundamental hereditary material found in all cells. Its hereditary function is based on two properties: (1) its ability to be exactly replicated and (2) its capability for transfer of its hereditary information to other biological molecules. Both properties depend upon its relatively simple but remarkable structure. It is an extremely long threadlike molecule whose subunits are linked by a single type of chemical bonding. There are only four kinds of subunits, designated A, T, C, and G, any one of which may be linked to any other in assembling the thread. The sequence of the subunits is the basic genetic information; for example, CATTACTTAGGT contains five recognizable words—cat, at, tact, act, and tag. In actual genetic language, however, only one of these "words" would be "read" because the genetic code involves triplets in sequence. Hence CAT, TAC, TTA, and GGT are the significant combinations, only the first of which happens also to be a meaningful word. In genetic language, however, all four are meaningful, each specifying an element of a protein.

DNA usually occurs biologically not as a single strand but as two strands wound around each other in a unique way. Binding between the two strands depends upon a second kind of chemical interaction between the subunits, in this case highly selective; C always is bound to G, and A to T. Thus the second *complementary* strand to that written above must be GTAATGAATCCA. It is this complementary relation between the two strands that makes

DNA replicable. If the strands are separated under suitable conditions, including the availability of free subunits, each subunit of each chain will bind its complementary subunit. Thus two double chains will result, identical in sequence to the first double chain. The essential *sequence* that constitutes the hereditary information can thereby be replicated, and is so replicated in every reproductive event.

Since the subunit sequence is so important and is so carefully preserved, it may be expected that any change will have genetic and developmental consequences. That is indeed the case. Change of a single subunit can yield crippling disease, as in the case of human sickle cell anemia. Such changes are as faithfully replicated as the original sequence—hence the hereditary nature of the disease. Changes of sequence of greater magnitude may also occur, particularly when breakage of strands is followed by repair with a long sequential piece in a new position. This is what occurs in recombination, whether natural or artificially induced, and such processes are the basis for recombinant DNA technology.

Proteins, particularly those that function as enzymes, not only are the recipients of the genetic information borne by DNA but also are essential to its replication and transfer of information. Certain proteins cut DNA strands at particular subunit sequences; others act to repair the breaks. By using such enzymes appropriately on purified DNA, it is possible to break and rejoin DNA from entirely different sources—for example, from a virus and a mammalian cell. A recombinant virus can thus be produced that carries mammalian genetic information. If the virus infects a mammalian cell and reproduces within it, it will replicate not only its own DNA but the included mammalian DNA as well. Since viruses often become incorporated into the chromosomal DNA of their host, they can act as a *vector* to introduce new mammalian genetic information into a mammalian cell. If the introduced DNA is of known biological significance and is expressed by making its characteristic product, this technique becomes a powerful one for controlled alteration of hereditary characteristics.

Consider the following recently reported experiment on adult mice (18). One of the persistent limitations in human cancer therapy is that both radiation and chemotherapeutic agents affect not only tumors but also such normally proliferating tissues as bone marrow, intestinal cells, and hair follicles. Bone marrow is especially important, since its cell products are essential to resistance to infection. Methotrexate is a widely used chemotherapeutic agent whose dosage has to be limited because of its side effects on normal cells. Certain mice, however, show a genetically determined resistance to methotrexate in their bone marrow cells. The question is raised whether this resistance could be transferred to other mice so as to protect them against higher methotrexate dosages required to control tumors.

The experiment involved extraction of DNA from methotrexate-resistant mice. Bone marrow cells of non-methotrexate-resistant mice were grown in culture in the presence of the methotrexate-resistant DNA. The cells were then reinjected into their donors, which were being maintained on a low methotrexate dosage. It is known that reinjected bone marrow cells will recolonize the bone marrow. In this instance, given the methotrexate dosage being maintained, only methotrexate-resistant cells would be expected to survive. In fact, 70 to 80% of the injected animals became methotrexate-resistant, a result that suggests that recombination had introduced the methotrexate-resistant gene into the treated cells.

If successfully applied to humans, this procedure could importantly improve cancer chemotherapy. However, there is a further possible application suggested by the investigators. Sickle cell anemia results from a genetic defect in globin, the protein portion of the respiratory pigment hemoglobin. The globin gene has been isolated and has been shown to function on incorporation into mammalian cells. If the globin gene could be combined with the methotrexate-resistant gene, then if methotrexate resistance was conferred on an individual afflicted with sickle cell anemia, normal hemoglobin production might be conferred as well. In other words, the anemia might be corrected by a gene insert, an example of therapy by genetic intervention.

This would be a medical milestone and something very like it is already reported in press accounts to have been attempted, although without success. It is important to recognize, however, that this would be genetic intervention, but it would not alter hereditary behavior in the usual sense of transmission between generations. This is how the window opened by external fertilization becomes relevant. When ordinary cells of the body (somatic cells) are altered genetically, as they are believed to be in cancer, their descendant *cells* are altered, but not the descendant offspring of the whole organism. This is because sperm and eggs are produced from a special cell population set aside early in development, the germ line consisting of primitive germ cells. Only genetic modifications of these cells can appear in offspring. Clearly, then, to produce genetic modifications transmissible between generations, one must alter cells of the germ line or introduce into it cells of an extraneous type that can function as germ line cells.

Precursors to the germ line, as to all cell types, are the early cleavage cells and the inner cell mass to which they give rise. Successful incorporation of recombinant DNA into these cells might induce genetic change transmissible through generations. This has not been demonstrated to occur regularly in any complex organism, and technical difficulties may negate the possibility. Nonetheless, the experiment is being attempted in mice for both its fundamental and its practical interest. If it succeeds, a rationale for its possible application to humans would be to assure healthy children to couples, both of whom are carriers for the same defective gene—for example, sickle cell anemia. It is not likely, certainly for a long time to come, to be useful for influencing such genetically complex characteristics as stature, personality, or intelligence.

To summarize this chapter, we have seen that advancing developmental knowledge, particularly about the mouse, is providing information and procedures for modifying fundamental aspects of reproduction, heredity, and development. In human terms, the new accessibility of the early human embryo affords options for applying this information and these procedures medically and, conceivably, for other benefits. A number of these possibilities raise significant ethical, social, and political issues. We shall turn to these in the next chapter.

GENERAL REFERENCES

Austin, C. R. (ed.), *The Mammalian Fetus in Vitro*. London: Chapman & Hall (1973).

Balls, M., and Wild, A. E., *The Early Development of Mammals*. New York: Cambridge University Press (1975).

Biggers, J. D., and Borland, R. M., Physiological aspects of growth and development of the preimplantation mammalian embryo. *Ann. Rev. Physiol.* **38**: 95–119 (1976).

Ciba Symposium, *Embryogenesis in Mammals*, No. 40 (NS). Amsterdam: Elsevier (1976).

Ciba Symposium, *The Freezing of Mammalian Embryos*, No. 52 (NS). Amsterdam: Elsevier (1977).

Daniel, J. C., *Methods in Mammalian Reproduction*. New York: Academic Press (1978).

David, I. B., and Wahlz, W., Application of recombinant DNA technology to questions of developmental biology: A review. *Develop. Biol.* **69**: 305–328 (1979).

Grobstein, C., *A Double Image of the Double Helix: The Recombinant DNA Debate*. San Francisco: Freeman (1979).

Johnson, M. H. (ed.), *Development in Mammals*, Amsterdam: Elsevier/North Holland (1978).

Karp, L. E., and Donahue, R. P., Preimplantational ectogenesis: Science and speculation concerning *in vitro* fertilization and related procedures. *Western J. Med.* **124**: 282–298 (1976).

Martin, G. R., Teratocarcinomas and mammalian embryogenesis. *Science* **209**: 768–776 (1980).

McLaren, A., *Mammalian Chimeras*. New York: Cambridge University Press (1976).

New, A. C., Mammalian embryos during organogenesis. *Biol. Rev.* **53**(1): 81–122 (1978).

Russell, L. (ed.), *Genetic Mosaics and Chimeras in Mammals*. New York: Plenum: (1978).

Sherman, M. I., and Solter, D., *Teratomas and Differentiation*. New York: Academic Press (1975).

Sherman, M. I., *Concepts in Mammalian Embryogenesis*. Cambridge: MIT Press (1977).

Chapter IV

Sorting the Issues

In this chapter we shall survey certain of the issues raised in hearings on external human fertilization conducted by the Ethics Advisory Board of the Department of Health, Education and Welfare. The Board was asked by then Secretary Joseph Califano to examine the scientific, ethical, legal, and social issues surrounding external human fertilization and embryo transfer in general (Appendix I). The Board responded with a six-month study in which it commissioned reports by scholars and experts in relevant areas, held eleven public meetings in various parts of the country, and received over 2000 pieces of correspondence bearing on the issues. The Board's report was formally released on May 9, 1979 (Appendix II), along with an appendix containing the reports of the commissioned experts and other documentation. This chapter draws heavily on these materials.

The study turned up a veritable thicket of questions and concerns. LeRoy Walters, Director of the Center for Bioethics of the Kennedy Institute at Georgetown University and a Special Consultant to the Board, dissected the tangle into individual issues and collated expert opinions on each (19). However, Leon R. Kass, one of the experts who prepared a commissioned paper and who has written extensively on the matter over the years, observed that "there is a latent danger of overlooking the forest for the trees in the otherwise rational procedure of considering the issues one at a time" (20). It is true that some of the character and force of an interrelated set of issues may be lost in an analytical process. On the other hand, the individual issues are too numerous and varied to be presented effectively as a random series. There are, in fact, several major themes around which the issues cluster. The first is the technical aspect, including such questions as whether there is a demonstrable and legitimate need, whether the procedure is within acceptable risk, whether it is efficacious, and whether there are options of comparable advantage. This aspect has been touched on in earlier chapters and will be returned to in the last.

A second group of issues bears on aspects of human nature and on human purposes and aspirations. These will be covered largely in this chapter, but with greater detail on a central issue in this category in the next chapter. A third grouping may be called sociopolitical issues. They will be reserved for the last chapter.

A Basic Human Pentad

Any discussion of human nature must recognize a set of basic attributes that are strongly linked and that represent an important foundation of human culture. These attributes are frequently referred to in discussions of external human fertilization as matters on which the procedure has likely impacts. As a group they span the biological, behavioral, and social realms, constituting a kind of slope between animal and human states along which our species has moved evolutionarily and continues to cycle generationally. The set includes sexuality in the biological sense, behavioral and social interactions between the sexes, childbearing and parenting, marriage, and family. I shall refer to this set as the "basic human pentad." A number of issues discussed in relation to external human fertilization can be best considered against the background of the pentad and its linkages.

The existence and significance of the pentad is not contested by the fact that it varies in its stability and force at different times, in different societies, and in different cultural niches. Nor has its importance been reduced by the notable shifts in attitudes toward it in the United States in recent years. In fact, the fierce controversies generated by the shifts in its linkages only emphasize the deep-lying meaningfulness of both the elements and their relationships, both to the contestants and to the whole culture. The vehemence of attack and defense reflect the high tension and emotion engendered by change, whether of degree or quality, in the overall relatedness of these five profound human experiences.

At the very core of the pentad are the biological phenomena of internal fertilization and internal gestation. Consider that this way of forming new generations was already long in existence in our ancestry when human culture first began. Internal genesis of the young is as central to the basic human pentad as the kitchen and its hearth are central to the primordial home. Consider, also, that the necessary natural prelude to internal genesis is sexual intercourse, one of the most strongly motivated human behaviors. Our premonitions concerning this, our experiences, dreams, and recollections, dominate much of our individual lives and strongly color our social behavior. Internal gestation, likewise, is deeply influential, certainly on women, not insignificantly on men, and in an uncertain degree on the early development of both sexes.

Around this highly charged mélange orbit human sexual roles and behavior, spousal love, the institution of marriage, the conception and care of children, and the establishment of family. The basic human pentad must have been importantly shaped by the existence of internal fertilization and gestation in the earliest human antiquity.

In no way, therefore, can the sudden displacement of so primordial a process be treated as a simple translocation in space from internal to external. The wrench is epic in human history. However cleverly biological consequences may be technically minimized, the translocation cannot fail eventually to generate profound emotional, cultural, and social reverberations. The immediate effect reminds one of the old trick of snapping a tablecloth off a finely set dinner table. Nothing else may move, but an essential feature, a unifying element of the tableau, has suddenly been snatched away. The potential sequel is suggested by the story about the infinitely sharp knife whipped through the neck of a victim of an execution. The victim merely blinks and then exclaims, "Ha, you never touched me!" "Wait," says the executioner, "until you turn your head!"

Strong reactions, including deep concern, are therefore not unexpected responses from those who confront for the first time the stark fact that the earliest and, in significant ways, the most vulnerable stages of human life now lie at least partly exposed to observation and, potentially, to manipulation. There are imaginable consequences of great magnitude, particularly its impacts on the basic human pentad. This is the contextual envelope for the several more discrete issues that, within the envelope, form a tangled, net-like skein. We shall take up these individual, though interacting, issues now in that context.

The Issue of Unnaturalness

LeRoy Walters (19) refers to the matter of unnaturalness as a presupposition of the debate over external human fertilization. I presume him to mean by this that many people take one side or the other as a "given," not subject to debate. He points to three identifiable positions that have been taken: (1) "Natural reproduction is inherently superior in a moral sense"; (2) "artificial methods can be justified when natural reproduction is impossible"; and (3) "artificial methods of reproduction are inherently superior." Another logically possible position is that the distinction between artificial and natural is overdrawn and that neither is superior *a priori*, either ethically or practically.

Walters quotes Kass (21) as a strong proponent of the first position: "Is there possibly some wisdom in that mystery of nature which joins the pleasure of sex, the communication of love, and the desire for children in the very activity by which we continue the chain of human existence?" And, again, "the laboratory production of human beings is no longer *human* [italics in original] procreation . . . making babies in laboratories—even "perfect" babies—means a degradation of parenthood."

At the opposite extreme, Walters quotes Joseph Fletcher (22): "Should we leave the fruits of human reproduction to take shape at random, keeping our children dependent on the accidents of romance and genetic endowment, of sexual lottery or what one physician calls 'the meiotic roulette of his parents' chromosomes'? Or should we be responsible about it, that is, exercise our rational and human choice, no longer submissively trusting to the blind worship of raw nature?"

In examining the issue, we cannot take for granted that all are agreed on what "natural" means. Is it the way things are without human interventions or contamination by human artifice? If so, it has a good, clean sound; it seems simple and idyllic. But it implicitly assumes that we humans are not natural but something apart.

This is difficut to reconcile with what we know about ourselves, our origins, our exchanges with and dependence on the nonliving and the rest of the living world. Yet, if we are ourselves part of the natural world, how can our intervention in any natural process make it unnatural?

Leaving conundrums aside, note that, although internal fertilization clearly is a step in the natural human process of reproduction, artifice frequently has been introduced in the form of contraception, artificial insemination, and sexual aids. External fertilization certainly goes beyond the internal equivalent in the introduction of artifice but does not totally supplant natural processes. Artifice is introduced to bring egg and sperm together and to insert the developing embryo into the uterus. But fertilization itself occurs naturally, as does cleavage and, subsequent to reinsertion, implantation in the uterine wall.

Nonetheless, this difference in degree is significant and offends the sensibilities of many people. In their view these are matters to be left to nature's way, either because of taboo or because nature's way is believed to be superior to any human artifice. Paul Ramsey, Professor of Religion at Princeton University and specialist in social philosophy and Christian ethics, is one of the strongest opponents of external human fertilization. In his presentation to the Ethics Advisory Board he emphasized especially the necessary uncertainties with respect to possible damage to offspring. Having described these, as he sees them, he told the Board that "no woman should have wanted a baby under these stated conditions . . . nor should any such thing ever be approved by the Ethics Advisory Board. Only an unexamined preference for *human design* over nature can support any other conclusion" (italics in original) (23). Clearly, Professor Ramsey has greater confidence in nature than in human design; he sees the two as opposites and would discourage if not prohibit the unnatural.

Unnaturalness or artificiality itself, however, does not seem to be entirely the crux of the matter. There are few objections to mechanical limbs, or to glass eyes, or to reconstructive surgery that often includes implantation of artificial materials. There has been little public outcry against efforts even to design artificial hearts. What is seemingly most objectionable is artificiality in the *generative function* itself, artificiality that affects procreation and allows it to be separated from sexual behavior. Yet contraceptives allow sexuality without procreation, and, increasingly, our mores have sanctioned sexuality without marriage.

The crux of the issue of naturalness appears to lie not so much with artificiality per se as with the consequent accessibility of the generative process to manipulation and the implications this has for the basic human pentad. As comes through clearly in Kass' comment quoted above, external fertilization is another threat of change in the linkages within the pentad and in attitudes toward them. Thus, Professor Ramsey speaks of "the *immediate* and not uninvited assault this procedure brings against marriage and the family" (24).

On the other side, it is to be noted that the pentad already is being reshaped and that external fertilization, in the context of its presently defined therapeutic purpose, is hardly likely to become a final engine for total destruction of the pentad or its linkages. On the contrary, the immediate purpose is to provide a child and create a family, an objective exactly opposite to the concern expressed. Nonetheless, it is true that external fertilization opens options that may go well beyond alleviation of spousal infertility. Some of these options, if chosen, could put further stress on the pentad. These options, it should be said again, arise not so much out of artificiality itself as out of the accessibility of the externalized egg and early embryo. We shall say more of this later.

The Issue of Descent

Descent refers to genetic transmission between generations, a purely biological phenomenon. It does, however, also evoke important psychological and social overtones. In internal fertilization, one can be certain that both parents have made a genetic contribution to the child. It is in that sense the couple's own, by genetic descent. No one who has listened to endless discussions about whom a child resembles most, sometimes going back several generations, can fail to appreciate the intense interest that centers on genetic linkage within families. The issue to be discussed is the degree to which external fertilization is likely to disrupt or weaken either the fact or the sense of descent and lineage.

In the case of external fertilization involving spouses, there seems little ground for concern with respect to the *fact* of descent. The genetic linkage between the generations is established at fertilization regardless of the site of the event. The externally fertilized egg is exactly as much the genetic descendant of the parents as is the internally fertilized one. However, the *sense* of descent is another matter. It needs consideration with respect to both parents and offspring. The possibility cannot be excluded that certain parents might feel differently about an offspring conceived in an incubator following separate manipulations performed on the two of them. Lack of the experience of physical union at the time of conception could be a significant factor psychologically. It can also be argued, conversely, that the special efforts to ensure a conception should lead to greater, not lesser, emotional attachment. These are matters for careful attention in the selection of candidates for the procedure and for continuing professional counseling in the event of success. The problem is not different in principle and seems less severe than that faced in adoption.

Possible effects upon the offspring are more difficult to assess. There can at the moment only be speculation, since it is too early for information on the few successful cases reported. Experience with adoption again is relevant, although the two situations have important differences. The best one can say is that the unusual nature of the conception is one more factor to be taken into account in sensitive child-rearing. Professional advice should be available and may be increasingly helpful to both parents and children as experience accumulates.

The descent issue becomes more complex if nonspousal external fertilization is admitted. This matter has been extensively discussed by Kass who expresses great concern. He suggests that "clarity about who your parents are, clarity in the lines of generation, clarity about who is whose, are the indispensable foundations of a sound family life, itself the sound foundation of civilized community. Clarity about your origins is crucial for self-identity, itself important for self-respect. It would be, in my view, deplorable public policy further to erode such fundamental beliefs, values, institutions and practices" (25). Kass recognizes that many of the confusions he fears already exist as a result of artificial insemination, pregnancy out of wedlock, other forms of sexual promiscuity, high divorce rates, etc. Nonetheless, his concern is that the pentad will be further undermined, and he recommends particularly against any action that will promote nonspousal external fertilization.

Kass' case appears to rest more on his feeling that traditional linkages within the pentad represent eternal verities than on objective evidence that there are not other forms of linkage in other life styles that might be equally viable and satisfying. As matters move forward, it will be important to keep his caveats in mind. It is not inconceivable, however, that adjustments over time will make for very different judgments a generation or two hence.

Respect for Humanness

A third issue bearing on the basic pentad is the question of whether external fertilization is somehow disrespectful to the concept of humanness. It is a concern founded in a desire to preserve the special qualities of the human species relative to other forms of life. Belief in the special qualities of humanity can claim considerable support from comparative studies of humans and their nearest biological neighbors. Although there are many similarities at the biological level, there is evident discontinuity—for example, in capacity for language, cognition, sense of future, and purpose. Valuing this difference leads to resistance to intervention in and manipulation of the process of creation of a new human being. The suggestion is that, if human fertilization can be externalized and manipulated in much the same fashion as in frogs, mice, or cattle, this tends toward denigration of characteristic human qualities and may lead to brutalization of the species.

Once again, the ultimate effect is feared to be on the pentad. If fertilization, whether internal or external, becomes too clearly a totally biological process, this baser element may subvert the loftier ones of the pentad—conjugal love, the miracle of creation, the presumed selfless bonding of mother to child. To the degree that the pentad stabilizes higher social phenomena—community, respect for law, loyalty to country—all these may come crumbling down. In this sense, external fertilization, by biologizing the species, is seen as threatening essential human qualities that support a stable social order.

Needless to say, there is a countervailing view. To give aid and comfort to the afflicted is one of the higher manifestations of human quality; external fertilization is but a means to that end. To intervene in the process of fertilization is neither denigrating nor demeaning because fertilization itself is, first and foremost, a biological process. It is the union of two cells, albeit special ones, and in a special context clearly evident at psychological and social levels. There is no reason why external union cannot be carried out with appropriate respect and reverence; the oviduct is dark and inaccessible but endowed with no particular sanctity. It is not the site but the manner in which the phenomenon is viewed that protects the dignity of human fertilization.

Playing God

The unnatural aspects of external fertilization, our sensitivity about preserving recognizable lines of descent, and the importance of respect for human dignity are all matters of deep concern to dominant religious faiths. Expressive of this concern is reference to interventions in human procreation as "playing God." The implication is that human intervention in the creation of new lives is usurpation of the role of God, whose creative hand is seen as governing all of genesis.

The phrase has impact beyond the religious context. The concept of God includes the notion of omniscience. Any act of God implicitly is taken in full knowledge of all consequences. Such complete foreknowledge is rarely within human capacity. Consequently, most human decisions are taken in the face of significant uncertainty. The farther down the road one attempts to forecast consequences, the greater the uncertainty. The term "playing God," used pejoratively, implies that we are making Godlike decisions without Godlike omniscience. If we know not what we do, we might be headed for severe trouble.

The human approach to this kind of situation has always been pragmatic. Human beings have been intervening in procreation in other species—also scripturally God's work—for a long time. To a lesser degree, we have also been intervening in our own procreation, with increasing reliability. A new dimension in such intervention is now being achieved, with external fertilization an outcome of earlier interventive capabilities and a clear harbinger of more to come. But should the earlier steps not have been attempted because the present ones might be their consequence? Should the economic advantages of artificial insemination in cattle be forgone because the knowledge gained might be applied to humans? The fact is that human artificial insemination has neither displaced the natural process nor, despite certain unresolved questions, produced obvious deleterious effects when carried out for socially acceptable purposes.

What is now happening with external fertilization, it can be argued, is dramatized but not clarified by invoking comparison with acts of God. To seek to understand and then to apply this understanding to human problems has always been and remains the human way. Given socially acceptable purpose, responsible human beings do not avoid all foreseeable risk, let alone succumb to fear of speculative risk. They proceed sequentially by probing consequences as far into the future as possible, making the appropriate decision for the time, and assuming that a later decision will be better informed by the knowledge that greater experience will bring. This is not playing God; it is being human, often in areas that previously were subject to religious or other taboos that entered tradition during a less knowledgeable time.

The Slippery Slope

But this last argument is exactly the one that some people fear. They foresee a series of steps, each one justified by the assertion that it is only a small change from the one that went before, yet yielding a new benefit, whether it be a practical one or one of greater understanding. Thus, we may begin with the most acceptable case—external fertilization between spouses to alleviate female infertility—but quickly proceed to the converse case of male infertility. Infertility in men often is the result of a low sperm count in the ejaculate. It takes only a single sperm for actual fertilization of the egg, but many millions of sperm have to be introduced into the vagina to guarantee that sufficient numbers will reach the egg to ensure that one will penetrate. A normal male ejaculate has a sperm count ranging from 50 to 60 million per milliliter. With counts below 20 million per milliliter, males usually are infertile. Clearly there is very heavy dilution and attrition of sperm as they spread upward in the female genital tract. In external fertilization, however, only about 50,000 sperm are needed to ensure that one sperm will penetrate the egg. Therefore, it clearly is possible that a male who is infertile in the normal internal process may be fertile in the external one. The likelihood can be increased by centrifuging a semen sample to increase the sperm density.

External fertilization to assist infertile males has not yet been reported. However, the first fertility clinic in the United States to announce its intention to use external fertilization reportedly intends to test the possibility. This would be a step along the slippery slope, because, instead of the egg donor being herself sterile, she presumably would be normal and yet would bear the burden of inconvenience and possible risk. Since the procedure would not be to correct any defect in her but rather that of her husband, it would be one step further from the usual medical criterion that intervention is for the benefit of the immediately afflicted. If this step is sanctioned, it would take only a small additional step for a normal woman to donate eggs for other purposes—for example, following spousal fertilization to be implanted into another woman's uterus because her ovary has been removed.

Further progressions along the slippery slope can be envisioned from our earlier discussion of procedures that have been successful on mouse eggs and embryos. They can be collectively characterized as reproductive, developmental, and genetic intervention deliberately practiced on the human species to meet human needs and purposes. Kass, in his testimony to the Ethics Advisory Board, left no doubt as to his own expectations about progression along the slippery slope. He projected "at least the following" (26):

1. Growth of human embryos in the laboratory beyond the blastocyst stage. Kass conceded uncertainty as to how far

this might go but did not exlude the possibility of "full-term ectogenesis."

2. Attempts to alter "the cellular and genetic composition of these embryos," including chimera formation, nuclear transplantation, cloning, and insertion of recombinant DNA.
3. Storage and banking of living human eggs and embryos.

Kass referred to the multiple questions such developments would raise but turned away from their detailed discussion to "serious objection to considering them at all." He argued that the logic used to justify even spousal external human fertilization was equally cogent for all that might follow. "This logic knows no boundary at the blastocyst stage, or for that matter at any later stage," he said. He warned the Board that "in the decision it must now make (it) may very well be helping to decide whether human beings will eventually be produced in laboratories." "Once the genies let the babies into the bottle," he said, "it may be impossible to get them out again." Kass recommended against federal funding for any research on human external fertilization or for the culture or transfer of human embryos because, among other reasons, "it will be difficult to forestall dangerous present and future applications of this research and its logical extensions." In short, he recommended against taking the first step onto the slippery slope.

Paul Ramsey (27) came to similar conclusions with somewhat different emphases. "*In vitro* fertilization and embryo transfer should not be allowed by medical policy or public policy in the United States—not now, not ever." He called upon all concerned to "take appropriate action to the extent of their jurisdictions to stop embryo manipulation as a form of human genesis." He finds "*conclusive* [italics in original] reasons for not continuing these experimental trials and for not allowing the procedure to become standard practice in the United States." Among his reasons were what he regards as *immediate* (italics in original) prospects for extension of the external fertilization technique far beyond its current purpose.

Samuel Gorovitz (28) challenged the slippery slope argument head-on. Using his perspective as a skier, he noted that it is possible to make judgments about which slippery slopes one can handle and which one cannot. Moreover, it is not the case that entry onto a particular slippery slope implies that one must go all the way or crash at the bottom. "It is a question of control and, in part, of judgment." He then proceeded to consider the slippery slope argument in relation to external human fertilization. He noted that the position taken by both Kass and Ramsey assumes the absence of judgment and control and, therefore, a progression down the slope to the ultimate imaginable consequence—for example, full human ectogenesis and destruction of the family. He argues that "there is no reason to take such a position seriously. Collectively, we do have a significant capacity to exercise judgment and control." It is not the case that, in liberalizing abortion laws to allow the killing of fetuses, in deference to maternal rights, we have gone on to sanction infanticide. "A process of social policy determination has exercised judgment," not necessarily making everyone happy but demonstrating that "we can stop a process once we have begun it." In accord with his treatment of the slippery slope argument, Gorovitz' recommendations would sanction research at early stages of human development, but not later, for reasons to be discussed further on.

As both Kass and Gorovitz note, the crux of the slippery slope argument is really the implicit or stated rationale for proceeding or not proceeding with external human fertilization research and clinical application. If the rationale is to alleviate infertility in marriage due to obstructed oviducts in a wife, than no sanction is given for any, even small, further development. If the rationale is to alleviate infertility in general, then sanction is given not only for nonspousal application but for recovery of eggs from normal women in order to compensate for infertility in their husbands. The choice is one of purpose. Spelling that purpose out clearly defines how long and steep a slope we are on and how far along it we are willing to go. To accomplish such clarification is the function of policy debate and decision. In making the decision, a precise rationale must be specified in order to identify the slope it puts us on and to determine how far we are currently willing to proceed before engaging in a new debate and decision. We shall return to this important matter in the last chapter.

Rights of the Developing Embryo

In what are regarded as enlightened societies, individual members are guaranteed a number of rights. These are protective assurances by the society against untoward happenings to its members. They are of various kinds, depending upon the value systems of the society. Among the most fundamental and universal rights are protection of life, protection against mutilation or torture, and protection against intervention in or invasion of the person without informed consent. Impugnment of these rights is raised as an issue by external human fertilization, as it has been by abortion. The crux of the issue is when in the course of development these rights apply.

In relation to abortion, the United States Supreme Court (29) has ruled that the rights of the mother take precedence over the rights of the developing offspring in her uterus. This makes clear that the rights of the developing offspring are not equal to those of an adult, but it does not address the question of what rights the embryo has—either at different stages of development or, in the special case raised by external fertilization, when it is external to the mother and no conflict of rights is involved.

A variety of positions has been taken on the matter, in scholarly and public discussion and before the Ethics Advisory Board. They range from assignment of full rights from the moment of conception to denial of any rights up to the moment of birth and the achievement of independent respiration. In societies that practice infanticide, rights are not accorded until some stage of external maturation. In our own society it has been suggested that right to life should not be accorded until some 48 hours after birth in order to assess the state of the newborn and to give opportunity to terminate lives with poor expectancy for acceptable quality. The suggestion has found little support, and infanticide for any reason, even in premature infants of dubious viability, is generally regarded as a violation of the right to life.

It is between the limits of conception and capability for semi-independent viability that opinions vary and controversy rages. LeRoy Walters (19) notes that in relation to the clinical aspects of external human fertilization the matter comes up particularly with respect to "discarded" early embryos. This may occur if the procedure involves superovulation and only a single embryo is selected for implantation, or if the embryo resulting from external fertilization is not judged to be certainly enough normal to risk transfer to the uterus. If right to life exists at this stage, failure to transfer any embryo to the uterus is a breach of that right, whether it be established ethically or legally. There is also a breach if a transferred embryo fails to develop normally and is aborted, either spontaneously or by induction.

If right to life is not established until some later stage, as the Supreme Court decision suggests (at least when embryo right is in conflict with maternal right), then the argument against external fertilization on the ground that it involves some discard and wastage of early embryos loses force. Gorovitz supported this view in testimony before the Ethics Advisory Board, arguing that "the onset of the capacity for sentience marks a qualitative change in the development of the fetus . . . . It is an empirical question of neurological development when that change occurs" (30). Were this position to be accepted, the question of rights of the developing embryo would not arise until it was well beyond the stages externalized during the clinical external fertilization procedure—since there is not even a recognizable precursor of the nervous system prior to implantation. This matter seems so fundamental to the whole debate over external human fertilization that it is the subject of the entire next chapter.

Whenever it should be decided that the embryo acquires rights, the question would still persist whether the whole external fertilization procedure violates these rights, since it is initiated at a time when the individual placed at risk does not exist in a form able to give informed consent. Precedent exists for informed consent by surrogate when individuals are unconscious or otherwise incapacitated for effective decision-making. Parental consent, under the circumstances of external fertilization, is subject to challenge as possibly involving conflict of interest, since the parents are the motivated parties and probably are unusually risk-tolerant. Some kind of third-party trustee as surrogate might be helpful, but would not remove the dilemma of responsibility in the event of birth of an abnormal child.

These considerations apply to the rights of an embryo intended to be implanted and, therefore, necessarily take into account the person-to-be. Under present circumstances an unimplanted human embryo can certainly not survive to become a person. What, then, are its rights? Must it be kept alive as long as possible? Can it, or must it, be destroyed? Can it be observed, manipulated, or experimented upon to contribute to knowledge? Does it come under the protection of the requirements for human experimentation? These are questions that have no answer in law at the moment and are viewed very differently by those with different value systems. They raise the fundamental issue of the genesis of humanness, as it is viewed biologically, behaviorally, and socially. We shall examine this issue in the next chapter.

GENERAL REFERENCES

Edwards, R. G., Fertilization of human eggs *in vitro*: Morals, ethics and the law. *Quart. Rev. Biol.* **49**: 3–26 (1974).

Fletcher, J., *The Ethics of Genetic Control: Ending Reproductive Roulette.* Garden City, New York: Anchor Books (1974).

Goodfield, J., *Playing God: Genetic Engineering and the Manipulation of Life.* New York: Random House (1977).

Kass, L. R., Making babies—the new biology and the "old" morality. *Public Interest* **26**: 18–56 (1972).

Kass, L. R., "Making babies" revisited. *Public Interest* **54**: 32–60 (1979).

Ramsey, P., *Fabricated Man: The Ethics of Genetic Control.* New Haven, Connecticut: Yale University Press (1970).

Ramsey, P., *Ethics at the Edges of Life.* New Haven, Connecticut: Yale University Press (1978).

U.S. National Commission for the Protection of Human Subjects of Biomedical and Behavioral Research, *Research on the Fetus: Report and Recommendations and Appendix.* Washington, D.C.: Department of Health, Education and Welfare (1975).

Watson, J., Moving toward clonal man: Is this what we want? *Atlantic* **227**: 50–53 (1971).

Chapter V

Becoming a Person

How, and even when, a person—a new human being—comes to be remains a considerable mystery. We cannot say, in terms of our own experience, when our sense of personhood, or self, began. Certainly it was before our earliest recollections as adults, and such recall does not extend back into the first several years of life in more than the dimmest way. Even less can be said of when the sense of self began in human evolution. It seems reasonable that it intensified during the early hominid stages a million or more years ago. The evidence with regard to experience of self by our nearest biological neighbors, the nonhuman primates, is suggestive but not conclusive. Some recently reported success in seeking communication with them can be interpreted to mean that somebody is there, but there is still controversy whether it is another self or merely an imitative reflection of our own self (31).

The problem, of course, is that we do not know what or where a person or a self *is* in any reliable objective way. The notion clearly is contained in such terms as I, ego, you, soul, mind, will, human being, individual, person. In its fullest development, as we know it in adult humans, self is aware, feels, thinks, imagines, reacts, and interacts socially. It is self that makes decisions, votes, has hopes, undergoes despair, exercises initiative and judgment, and has legal rights. Selfness is regarded as characteristically human, although we are hard put to draw a sharp line between the self we infer in other humans and the quasi-self that can be postulated in other species—particularly other mammals and especially primates. Nonetheless, it is the peculiarly human recognition, affinities, dependencies, and communications among selves that account for and powerfully bind human social groups, whether in marriage, family, community, nation, or world order.

Self and person overlap and for many purposes may seem identical. However, entertaining the possibility that chimpanzees and dogs have an inner world of self-awareness does not require that they be persons. A person is conceived as necessarily human, but self-awareness is at least imaginable in nonhumans. Whether self and body are one, two, or even three is debated among philosophers and scientists (32). Scientifically, we assume that self arises during the course of each human life, although a number of religions teach otherwise. But with all our scientific sophistication we have no certain measure, or even detector, of function of a *self* except in our own individual experience and in our recognition, through communication, of similar experiences in others. When we cannot *communicate* we are essentially deaf, blind, and dumb, whether it is a matter of becoming aware of another self or even of declaring our own.

Thus, in terms of the issues raised by external human fertilization and bitterly debated in connection with abortion, we cannot say with any reliability *exactly* when personhood appears in the course of development. We cannot even be sure what meaning to attach to the question. For we do not know whether the experience of personhood or self is single or composite. Certainly it can be fragmented and distorted by trauma, drugs, and both organic and psychological disease. Does it turn on like a light in development, or is its beginning more like painting a picture or writing a novel? When is enough completed to say that *it* exists?

Our ignorance sometimes embarrasses our capability to make coherent policy. There are ethical and legal questions for which more precise understanding of the concepts of human, person, and self are desperately important. Among these is the subject of this book, as we have seen in discussing some of the issues. In its fundamental abortion decision in 1973 (29), the United States Supreme Court commented: "We need not resolve the difficult question of when life begins. When those trained in the respective disciplines of medicine, philosophy and theology are unable to arrive at any consensus, the judiciary at this point in the development of man's knowledge is not in a position to speculate." Thus, although the personal experience of self is our deepest and most intimate sense of reality, the nature and origin of that experience remains obscure enough to intimidate justices, scientists, philosophers, and even theologians.

The obscurity is not due to lack of attention. Over the centuries few subjects have inspired more cogitation. There appears to be an inherent difficulty in the problem, partly the result of the complexity of the substrate of self and partly, perhaps, because it is self studying self. There clearly are special problems in achieving self-understanding—philosophically, scientifically, and in individual lives. Nor is it likely that the obscurity will be abruptly dispelled by any single discovery or stroke of insight. There probably is a long road ahead, a path of patient picking, dissecting, and reconceptualizing. It is even possible that self—standing at it does at the intersection of subjective and objective reality—will never be identically comprehended by the myriad selves who have and will experience it.

Yet some measure of consensus is essential, since the concept figures so prominently in everyday life, in fundamental philosophy, and in ethics, law, and politics. Indeed, there *is* a degree of practical consensus on certain aspects. A person, a self, is uniquely individual, and we have an uncanny knack for distinguishing and recognizing such individuality. Self is somehow continuous in a lifetime, despite great physical, biological, and psychological modification and change. Self is closely linked to interaction with others; an I and a you may be essential to emerging awareness of self. It is generally accepted, too, that at least the experience of self can be interrupted by sleep, injury, or anesthesia. Self and awareness of self are thus not identical, although no one knows what or where self is when it is not being aware. Perhaps related is the distinction made between the conscious and unconscious selves in the psychoanalytical concept of the inner determinants of behavior.

Preconditions for Self

In all this uncertainty, the particular difficulty that we must face is the time of origin of self in a single human life history. The objective is to put together what we do know about this scientifically. It is not, of course, to be assumed that the scientific perspective is the only significant one or that it can by itself solve the associated policy problems. It *is* assumed, however, that those who seek sound and humane policy will want to do so within the bounds of objectively verifiable knowledge.

As we have seen, it is now established that a human egg can be removed from a potential mother, fertilized by the sperm of a potential father in a laboratory dish, and returned to the uterus of the egg donor for successful development and birth. This involves "artificial" or technology-assisted initiation of a new self-genesis. The question has been raised whether the required manipulations of the egg, sperm, and fertilization product constitute illegitimate and immoral intrusion upon either an actual or a nascent self. The Ethics Advisory Board of the Department of Health, Education and Welfare has recommended (Appendix II) that, with certain provisos, the necessary manipulations not be regarded as illegitimate or immoral. What role did objectively verifiable knowledge play in this finding?

To answer this we should first say something about a typical course of biological development. The general term for development is genesis, the same word that has large and profound connotations in other contexts. It is associated with ancient origins and with legends of such great beginnings as that of the universe, of life in all its forms, and of the special life form that we call humanity. But, scientifically, genesis is not limited to origins that occurred in the past. It is equally applicable to origins that occur in the present or will occur in the future. Scientific genesis refers to the *processes* of becoming—whenever, wherever, and however these processes may occur. Thus, cosmic genesis refers to initiation, change, and the possible ultimate fates of the universe. In the biological world, which is relatively miniscule in relation to the cosmos, initiations and progressions go on endlessly. They are seen in generational turnover and in the beginnings and maturation of each new living organism. Continuing genesis is illustrated, for example, in the processes of egg initiation and maturation (oogenesis), in the process by which an embryo evolves from a fertilized egg (embryogenesis), and in the process of formation of a heart (cardiogenesis).

Each genesis flows continuously in time, but it is useful to distinguish several intergrading general stages: (1) *pregenesis*, when the necessary preconditions for an initiation are in place but initiation has not demonstrably begun; (2) *imminence*, when initiation has become so probable that it will shortly begin unless it is actively suppressed; (3) *primordium*, when initiation is demonstrable but little or nothing of the final stage is recognizable; (4) *maturation*, when the primordium is gradually acquiring the final properties; (5) *maturity*, when the final properties are present and stabilized.

Does the quality of self have some such genesis, as does the formation of a heart or a whole embryo? Or does the quality of self arise suddenly in a single step, without processes of becoming? The question is not trivial, because there are conceptions of self that exclude processes of genesis. After-life and reincarnation assume a persistence of something that is independent of biological generations. That something certainly is not clearly distinguishable from self. Such conceptions importantly influence public debate and policy and cannot be ignored in our kind of society. But scientific concepts cannot be ignored either. Their ability to generate consensus by appeal to objective experience can bring disputants to common ground. This is a great advantage when deeply divisive philosophical and religious values contend in a policy arena.

Does self, as we understand the matter scientifically, carry over from one generation to another? For human beings, in whom self is at least most characteristic and best developed, the answer must be unequivocally negative. In fact, this is exactly what a new generation means—that two selves contribute jointly to the origin of a new one. What *is* carried over from one generation to the next? Essentially, three things—life, human quality, and individuality. Let us be clear about each of these because ordinary language often intermixes them, as in the quoted opinion of the Supreme Court (p. V-76).

Self is not synonymous either with life or with human life. There is an abundance of life forms that have no self remotely comparable to that experienced by humans—bacteria, all plants, the less complex animals devoid of any semblance of a nervous system. Moreover, there is no question that life is continuous between generations and does not begin anew in each. Egg and sperm are alive, as is their fusion product. New life out of nonlife has not been created on the earth for at least some three billion years. All organisms are continuously living descendants from earlier ones. It is not life that begins in each human generation, it is self.

The same may be said of the quality of being human. Egg and sperm and their fusion product are each human, although it takes an expert to prove it. Size and shape, but most especially chemical composition, carry the indelible evidence of the human quality. Today we would say that the quality is found most consequentially in the chromosomal DNA, which is, in fact, the transfer agent from generation to generation. Thus, neither life nor the human quality begins in any generation. Human life, like that of all species, descends without break from generation to generation. It waxes and wanes in complexity but never begins *de novo*.

It is important to emphasize that the linkage between human generations is *cellular*, the lowest level of complexity at which human life can exist. The fusion-*cell* produced by fertilization is human life in a single cell. Descendant cells are *components* of an adult body that behaves as a whole human being. The properties by which we characterize and recognize the adult are not all present in the fusion-cell, although the capability to give rise to those properties during development *is* present. Self is a complex property of the adult, just as is the face or the bodily dimensions. When and how self begins in the developmental course is a question comparable to that of when and how the face begins. It is a separate question from that of human life, which does not begin at all in successive generations but is continuous between them.

Now what of the third carry-over element from generation to generation—individuality? Actually, individuality is not carried over intact; it is initiated in the fusion-cell by formation of a new *combination* of parental properties that *are* carried over. The sense in which this is a new individual has become a key issue. What is the nature of the new individuality in the fusion-cell, and what is its relation to the origin of self? To clarify this we must recognize two aspects of biological individuality—uniqueness and integralness. Uniqueness refers to the fact that the new individual has a vanishingly small chance of being identical with any other—on the earth or in the universe.

The uniqueness of each human zygote is genetic, arising out

of the sexual mechanism that underlies hereditary propagation in the human species. The hereditary mechanism includes the 46 chromosomes found in the nucleus of every typical human cell. As is well known, the chromosomes consist of 23 very similar but not identical pairs. The nonidentity of each pair stems from the fact that each parent contributes one chromosome to it. It is in this orderly fashion that the intimate and complex combination of parental contributions to offspring occurs.

The specific way in which parental contributions are combined can produce very rich genetic diversity (individuality) of offspring. This stems from a number of complexities in the way chromosomes behave during the formation of eggs and sperm. The progenitor cells for sperm and egg are typical in having 46 chromosomes in 23 pairs derived from the preceding generation (the grandparents). The sperm and egg have only 23 chromosomes, one from each pair. In each egg and sperm the pairs are represented independently in terms of their origin from mother and father. If we number the chromosomes in a particular sperm or egg, the first may be from the father, the second from the mother, the third from the mother, the fourth from the father, etc. The arithmetic of such a process says that a potential mother or father may produce 2^{23} genetically different eggs or sperm—8,388,608, or roughly 8.4th $\times 10^6$ of each. If these randomly combine in fertilization, we must square the number of possible kinds of eggs and sperm to determine the number of genetic kinds of offspring that a couple can produce—7×10^{13}. This diversity from a single couple already is 10,000 times as great as the number of humans currently on the earth, some 4×10^9. In fact, the additional complexities of chromosomal behavior in producing eggs and sperm makes the potential genetic variety far greater, for even a given couple, than that calculated on the basis of an independent assortment of chromosomes alone. The mechanisms of sexual hereditary transmission assure individual human uniqueness based upon genetic variety that is essentially infinite.

This endless genetic variety is the biological foundation for the unique individual that we associate with self, most especially our own self. A particular genetic combination, as it exists in chemical language in the chromosomes of the fusion-cell, is hardly equivalent, however, to the experiential and behavioral complexities by which we identify fully developed self. For example, a single fusion-cell, in twinning, may yield two genetically identical offspring, who are, nonetheless, physically and psychologically separate selves. Clearly, although genetic uniqueness is an important determinant of the individuality of self, it can hardly be equated with the complexity of its full expression. In the language of developmental genesis as outlined above, the establishment of genetic uniqueness corresponds only to pregenesis or, at most, to imminence.

Turning to unity or integralness as the second aspect of individuality, what has just been said about twinning makes it clear that the fertilized egg is not yet fixed as a *single* individual. It can give rise, under conditions that are not entirely understood in humans, to two identical twins. Experiments with eggs of other mammals show that even after the egg has divided several times its individual cells can still give rise to whole embryos. Conversely, embryos at the four-cell stage can be fused to produce a single individual. Integralness is, therefore, established not at fertilization but later in the developmental course.

Thus, the scientifically valid sense in which fertilization establishes a new individual can be stated as follows. When egg and sperm nuclei meet and fuse, a new and unique genetic constitution is established. This constitution may be expressed in one unitary individual, but it can be expressed under unusual circumstances in more or less than one. Fertilization therefore establishes a state of pregenesis with respect to a new individual by providing a unique new genome. This is a precursor but not equivalent to the integralness and eventual complexity of a new human being. The central problem scientifically is the nature of the transition from the pregenesis of a new self, established at fertilization to the full self-experience of the mature adult. Does self undergo a genesis along with that of other developing structures and functions? Parallel to this scientific problem is the policy question: At what stages in development do properties arise that should be accorded a level of legal and social rights, either as nascent or as realized selves?

The Imminence of Self

In these terms we may ask whether there is a stage of imminent self, a stage at which the probability that a self will be initiated is so high that only some degree of suppression will prevent it. Here the data on human embryo survival following *internal* fertilization are relevant. If, for the moment, we assume that a self in some form is present at birth, then among fertilized eggs there is a roughly one-in-three chance that a particular egg will give rise to a self (33). Following implantation, say at two weeks after fertilization, the probability that a particular surviving embryo will give rise to a new self has risen sharply; three out of four may be expected to do so. By six weeks, eight in ten will give rise to a new self, and by 18 weeks virtually all (97%) will do so. In these terms, imminence is relatively low in preimplantation stages, rises sharply following implantation, and achieves virtual certainty in late stages of pregnancy.

Recall, however, that imminence does not include the demonstrable presence of self. Abortion clearly suppresses self in some sense, the crucial question being at what stage it may terminate an actual self. External fertilization without insertion of the embryo into the uterus also results in suppression of at least imminent self, given our present inability to carry out complete ectogenesis. However, what we can presently say about the actual self-state of the embryo from the data we have been discussing is inconclusive. This is highlighted by the fact that if a human embryo were to be kept alive externally beyond the stage of implantation it would lose its state of imminence despite its continuing normal development, simply because we do not know how to maintain it externally to full term. We clearly need more cogent criteria for characterizing the self-status of developing embryos than their potential for completing development.

A Rudiment of Self?

Imminence can be put to use in studying many developmental processes. Having once detected an area of an embryo that will shortly and predictably begin to form a limb, one can more easily focus on the first steps in the process and then, by modifying or suppressing them in various ways, work out something about their significance. That approach, unfortunately, has little applicability to understanding the beginnings of self. We are forced to ask whether we can detect a later stage—that is, a rudiment of self. Here there is some information that may be helpful, at least in setting limits to the problem.

First, we must recall that if there were a rudiment of self it could not be recognized by looking for the characteristics of the mature state. The rudiment of a forelimb is not found by looking for a long bone like the humerus or for fingernails. The first sign that a forelimb is forming is an increased rate of cell division at the appropriate site. A localized difference in cell behavior marks the initiation of a limb. Correspondingly, if we are looking for a rudiment of self, we cannot expect to find recognition of a familiar face or a sense of loneliness. Such aspects of self probably do not exist even in a healthy newborn infant, and they certainly are not to be expected in a hypothetical rudimentary stage.

What might be expected? It seems reasonable that the most rudimentary and generalized aspect of self is simple sensation—for example, a feeling of comfortable warmth. The human embryo floats in a dark, fluid-filled chamber, normally at constant temperature. Its own developmental processes are gradually changing both it and the size and chemistry of the chamber it is in. At some point these changes within the embryo can be imagined to alter its state in a way that initiates a *feeling* of warmth. We should not, at this point, ask how this happens because, in truth, we do not know. All we can say is that it seems impossible to conceive of anything even approaching the experience of self that does not have *at least* such simple sentience.

Simple sensation, however, seems not enough to define a sense of self. To get at least one step closer there must be more than just diffuse, floating sensation. There must be some *thing* that is warm, there must be some center of feeling, there must be not only a sensate locus but a nonself surround. Self is not just sensation, it is sensation within a bounded object that is the physical equivalent of the discreteness of the feeling of self. A diffuse and unbounded sentience might be thought of as a nonindividualized preself, a bounded sentient *locus* as a rudimentary individualized self.

If such a rudimentary self-state existed, how could we recognize it? Not easily, given the fact that we normally depend upon communication to recognize another self. In the absence of communication we have to fall back on what may be called correlates of the feeling of self. These, as we distinguish them in relation to fully developed selfness, are, first, behavioral and, second, related functional processes. We accept as another self people who behave in certain ways or in whom it is possible to demonstrate functional processes that we judge to be closely involved in selfness. There is one other important consideration in assessing the self-state of developing humans. Although we directly know the experience of self only individually—as an internal state—we infer it in others and they in us. In the process, the sense of self is affirmed and reinforced. In that sense, self is partly a product of social interaction. In particular, the social status of personhood is accorded through recognition and acceptance by others. Recognition and empathy registered by observers are especially important criteria for assessing levels of selfness when policy issues are at stake. How much help can these several criteria provide in recognizing a rudimentary self-state?

Let us test this by applying the criteria to several stages of human development that have been or might be suggested to mark the beginning of a new human life, self, or person. The first is conception, the production of a fusion-cell by fertilization. We have already stated the biological significance of conception. It establishes a new genetic entity but does not immediately yield a first precondition for a new self—integralness. With respect to the criteria we have outlined for recognizing a rudiment of self, the fusion-cell certainly falls short. It shows neither behavior nor function that we associate with selfness, and it clearly is unrecognizable and generates no empathy in observers. The last statement has to be qualified. Some people who are expert, or who are informed that the object is a human fusion-cell, may experience a special kind of empathy based on their knowledge of the potential of the fusion-cell. The criterion, however, is intended to depend upon direct empathy with a recognizable and present other self, at least in a rudimentary state.

A second suggested stage for the initiation of a new human life, self, or person is implantation in the uterine wall. This clearly is an important step, since it initiates pregnancy in the mother, establishes the beginning of interactions that are so essential that the term maternal–fetal unit is applied, and marks a time when the probability of producing a fully developed new self rises markedly. By the three criteria suggested, however, the situation is little changed. As already noted, implantation produces heightened imminence but no evidence of a self-rudiment—behaviorally, functionally, or in recognition and empathy. In fact, if anything, the embryo at this stage loses identity, many of its cells merging almost indistinguishably into the maternal tissues. In rare, abnormal circumstances the embryo may actually lose *all* identity as a potential individual, becoming a hydatiform mole, a tumor that may threaten the life of the mother. In normal circumstances, however, relatively few cells of the embryo begin the process of formation of a new individual. To anyone but an expert these cells are unrecognizable, not only as a nascent self but even as an individual-to-be. Moreover, at this stage there is still a demonstrable capability in mice, which probably exists also in humans, to form two individuals (twinning) rather than one.

A third stage that may be considered is one to which a mammalian embryo has recently been carried externally. Compared with stages of conception and implantation, this is a fairly advanced state. The embryo proper is clearly recognizable within its membranes (Figure 5). It is, however, typically rudimentary in the sense in which we have defined the term. The major outlines of the future offspring can be discerned, but none of the properties of a mature state are yet present. The embryo is elongated, with a distinguishable head and tail end. One organ, the heart, although quite immature is functioning, pumping precursor blood through precursor vessels. The main axis of the body, eventually to be the spinal cord and the vertebral column, is demarcated by a series of rudiments—the somites—which are the source of later structures but do not themselves persist. A rudiment of the central nervous system is recognizable, expanded at the forward end as an indication of the beginning of formation of the brain. Were this a human embryo developing normally in the uterus, it would be in perhaps the sixth week following conception.

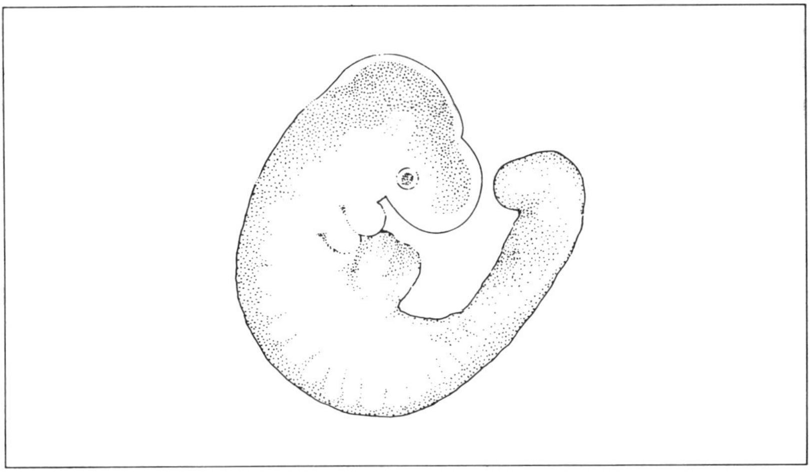

Figure 5. Advanced stage of mammalian (rat) development reached in laboratory culture. Note identifiable head and tail ends and such rudiments as somites, central nervous system, eye, jaw, and heart. (After photograph kindly supplied by D. L. Cockroft, Physiological Laboratory, Cambridge, England.)

What do our three criteria say of a rudimentary self possibly being present in a human embryo at this stage? The question forces us to return to our criteria and define them more fully. What, more precisely, do we mean by behavior diagnostic of a rudimentary self-state? What kind of behavior might be expected? Given a bounded sentience, what kind of output could it provide, if one assumes that behavior implies some output that can be externally registered? Minimally the output would be some kind of response to an external change. But if we require that, we are adding to our definition of a rudimentary self. It must not only be sentient and bounded, it must have some capacity for behavioral output. That is a part of what we rely on for diagnosis of more mature selves, but we may not want to admit it to our criteria for rudimentary selfness. Let us, for the moment, say only that in the stage we are considering there is no positive behavioral evidence of a rudimentary self. There simply is no behavior, in the usual sense of the term, either spontaneously or in response to any stimulus. Yet the absence of behavioral output does *not* assure us that a rudimentary sentient state may not be present.

What do we mean, more precisely, by the second criterion of nonbehavioral functional processes? In connection with adult self-states, reliance is placed almost entirely on functions of the nervous system. There is general consensus among scientists and philosophers who concern themselves with the nature of self that it is inextricably intertwined with activities and processes within the brain. The exact nature of these activities and processes cannot be specified, and it is likely to remain uncertain for some time, despite extensive research aimed at fathoming it. There is, however, growing information that sets limits on the circumstances under which selfness might be present.

One index is the significant electrical activity that can be detected by intracellular recording and by electroencephalography. Absence of electrical activity increasingly is the critical criterion for termination of self at death. A second is the degree of connection among nerve cells in the brain, especially in the cortex. Such connections become bewilderingly rich and complex but can be examined microscopically to provide an indication of brain maturation and, in some instances, of normality or abnormality of function. A third is the presence in functioning brain of specific substances that act as neurotransmitters—that is, mediate transfer of impulses from nerve cell to nerve cell. Normal brain function is inconceivable without these chemical intermediaries.

With this expanded meaning of the second criterion, the presence of a rudimentary self at the stage under consideration seems quite impossible. There is no demonstrable electrical activity characteristic of the nervous system. Microscopic examination indicates why. Although a *rudiment* of the nervous system can be identified, it shows, microscopically, none of the essential features for charcteristic function. The cells that make up the rudiment are still in rapid division and have not yet become nerve cells. There are no characteristic connections among them. Correspondingly, neurotransmitters have not yet appeared. If sentience depends upon any aspect of neural function, it cannot possibly yet be present. Whatever aspect of self is present at this stage, it must be less than the rudimentary state defined. If some aspect of self does exist at this stage, it is equally likely to be present in all living cells and organisms; it is not the *kind* of self that we experience so intimately and vividly.

Finally, by the third criterion of social recognition, this stage has also to be judged to be without a rudiment of self. A nonexpert has to be persuaded that there is anything recognizably human about the embryo, and even an expert will point out that most of its characteristics are the same as in monkeys, mice, birds, or even fish. This stage is, in fact, one fundamentally shared by all vertebrates. This, to emphasize again, is not to say that the embryo of this stage is not human. Like the fusion-cell, it is human in the deepest biological sense. But it has not yet acquired the recognizable social form of humanness.

Premonitions of Self

Let us now ask when in the course of human development signs appear suggesting, by the several criteria enumerated, that a rudiment of self *may* be present. It is these first signs that are important, on the assumption that under no circumstances would we wish to disrupt, interrupt, or impact upon the life of a self-aware human. We shall look first at behavior, second at functional capability, and third at social recognition. The question is which of these gives the earliest indication of need to confer some or all of the status, rights, and protections of personhood.

The earliest that responsiveness to stimuli has been reported in human embryos is at 7 to 8 weeks after conception (34). The embryos observed were delivered by caesarean section after a finding by a panel of obstetricians that termination of pregnancy was essential to maternal health. The delivered embryos were transferred promptly to a suitable mild salt solution maintained at body temperature. Cut off from placental circulation and too immature for independent survival, the embryos necessarily expired within a matter of minutes. But observations begun not more than two minutes after placental separation showed distinct responsiveness.

The embryos were stimulated by stroking the skin at various places with hairs carefully calibrated as to pressure exerted. The earliest responses were obtained by stimulation around the mouth at about seven weeks after conception. The response was a slow and weak turning of the head away from the stimulus, presumably resulting from stimulation of nerve endings in the skin. Judging from knowledge of later neurological connections, the nerve endings were probably those of fibers of the fifth cranial nerve, whose cell bodies are clustered near the brain. Head turning involves muscles of the neck. Therefore impulses coming in along the cranial nerve fibers must have been transferred within the central nervous system to other nerve cells having extensions going out to the neck muscles. The behavior indicates that at this stage some nerve cells are mature enough to transmit impulses and to transfer them from cell to cell. The behavior is a primitive, so-called "total pattern" reflex.

With older embryos, about 8 weeks from conception, the response was observed to become stronger and wider, eventually including movements not only of the head, but of the trunk, pelvis, limbs, and mouth. At still later stages, local rather than total pattern reflexes could be elicited that involved the limbs and other parts of the body.

What does this kind of reflex response imply with respect to sentience and selfness? The first answer must be that one cannot be sure. Clearly some degree of neural function is present, and it is not impossible that nerve cell and neurotransmitter activity always carries some degree of sentience. The second answer, however, is that other evidence gives no support to this interpretation and that the weight of all evidence, although not conclusive, appears to be against it. First, reflex responses of this general kind are stereotypic, "automatic"—quite different in flexibility and adaptiveness from the behavior normally associated with selfness. Second, responses of similar kind can be elicited in human adults who are unconscious and hence are not necessarily sentient. Third, such responses occur in nonhuman species—for example, in cats whose spinal cords have been severed above the level of stimulation and response. On the assumption that the brain is necessary for sentience (a reasonable but not necessary assumption on the evidence), simple reflexes involving only the cord do not indicate sentience. Fourth, in the human embryos of the stages tested by the procedures described, the spinal cord is far more mature neurologically than the brain. Adequate connections for spinal reflex activity can be demonstrated, but not for higher brain function.

Into the Gray Zone

A recent technical summary (34) of observations on exteriorized human fetuses suggests that "the reflex activities that have been demonstrated prior to 20 weeks of menstrual age [18 weeks postconception] are executed through the mesencephalon, the lower brain stem and the spinal cord and do not involve diencephalic or telencephalic centers." The reference here is to stages later than those described above and indicates that the lower brain (mesencephalon and lower brain stem) gradually becomes mature enough to function. The areas affected are also primarily involved with "automatic" activities—for example, regulation of heart rate, respiration, and other functions normally carried out even in adults without consciousness or volition. "After approximately 20 weeks," the summary continues, "neural circuits through the diencephalon and striatal complex (or basal ganglia) become functional in increasingly greater degree." These higher brain areas, particularly the striatal complex, are believed to play some role in arousal and hence conceivably in consciousness.

Even before 20 weeks, however, yet another new phenomenon appears—"spontaneous motility," movements that are not a response to any evident external stimulus. Slow, arrhythmic, asymmetrical, noncoordinated movements have been reported in exteriorized embryos as early as 9 to 10 weeks, and they become more pronounced with increasing maturity. Observations by ultrasonography (35) on fetuses *in utero* give evidence of movement at about this same time or possibly a little earlier. At about the tenth or eleventh week, movements become more distinct. They are described as being of two kinds—strong and brisk, or slow and sluggish. The strong and brisk movements are said to be "faintly reminiscent of the flapping motion" of the tail fin of a fish. As a result of the movement, the embryo, normally seen to rest at the bottom of the fluid-filled gestational sac, is projected upward; it floats down again after the movement is completed.

By 14 weeks, spontaneous movements of exteriorized fetuses are described as more coordinated and "graceful." At about 18 weeks, these and other movements are detectable to the mother—the traditional time of "quickening." The experience has been referred to as reminiscent of "fluttering of a bird in hand." The fetus grows rapidly beyond this point, with spontaneous movements that are increasingly noticeable to the mother and even to external observers.

These facts make it clear that spontaneous, as well as responsive, motility begins in the human fetus during the third month of gestation. Its occurrence can be correlated fairly closely with maturation of the biological substrate—that is, the appearance at the cell level of recognizable nerve cells, nerve endings, muscle fibers, and essential connections among them. Does "spontaneous" activity have greater implication for possible selfness than responsiveness? Again, there is no certain scientific answer. "Spontaneity" can be explained away as reflex responsiveness to unknown stimuli, whether from the outside or from changes of internal state. In fact, however, there is increasing evidence for self-generating neural centers in fairly simple behaviors requiring nothing comparable to a brain. The behavior described on the part of the early human embryo is not basically different from that commonly observed in young frog tadpoles that lie at the bottom of a dish and occasionally, for no apparent reason, erupt into vigorous swimming movements that carry them for some distance before they become quiescent and float back down to the bottom. The crucial question is whether such behavior implies some degree of sentience or even an active volition.

The consensus among scientists who study these behaviors and who express an opinion is that such behavior need not and probably does not require either sentience or selfness. The opinion is based largely on the degree of brain involvement and particularly on the probability of involvement of higher brain centers such as the cerebral cortex. For example, Carmichael (36) comments that "it is generally thought that even during the third month the cerebral cortex has as yet assumed no functions in relation to the general bodily activity." The comment is in accord with the continuing immaturity of the cerebral cortex well beyond the third month of human development.

The comment also is in accord with comparative observations of other organisms. Both spontaneous and responsive motility are shown by such relatively simple organisms as protozoa, hydroids, and flatworms. None of these organisms have a brain, and they are not *generally* regarded as possessing anything comparable to a self. More complex organisms, such as fish, frogs, and snakes, that do have a brain also show such a behavior. Their brains, however, have only weakly developed cortical areas, and they are not *generally* regarded as possessing a self. The problem becomes more difficult when mammals, especially nonhuman primates, are addressed. These animals have distinct cortical areas, although of smaller relative mass than that of humans. Their behavior is frequently such as to imply limited cognitive processes, and there is much controversy over their level of sentience and awareness. In recent years it has become clear (31) that chimpanzees can make and use tools, can develop language, and may be able to learn to communicate with humans by signing. They have also been reported to be self-aware, at least in the sense that they recognize themselves in a mirror and distinguish themselves from other chimpanzees. These facts suggest that both spontaneous and responsive motility, looked at phylogenetically, are not in themselves diagnostic of selfness. They may, however, be an early phase of a progression that leads to selfness.

Behavioral progression correlates with the relative size and the character of the organization of the cerebral cortex. If the same were true of human development, selfness could be absent, despite the seemingly self-oriented behavior, until the cortex and possibly other higher brain centers achieve some appropriate level of maturation (32, 37). It is clear that at the end of the third month the cerebral lobes are relatively small (little more than half of the brain mass), and the maturation of nerve cells has only barely begun. The relative mass of the cerebral lobes increases sharply during the second trimester, but the complex folding of the cortex that accompanies and permits its still greater enlargement does not occur until the third trimester (Figure 6). Moreover, it is in the third trimester that the interactive capability of cortical nerve cells appears to increase through complex branching of their processes and the appearance of rich, multiple connections among them (Figure 7). This increase continues well into postnatal life. Brain scientists who theorize about the material substrate of consciousness and self emphasize the number of cortical nerve cells and the

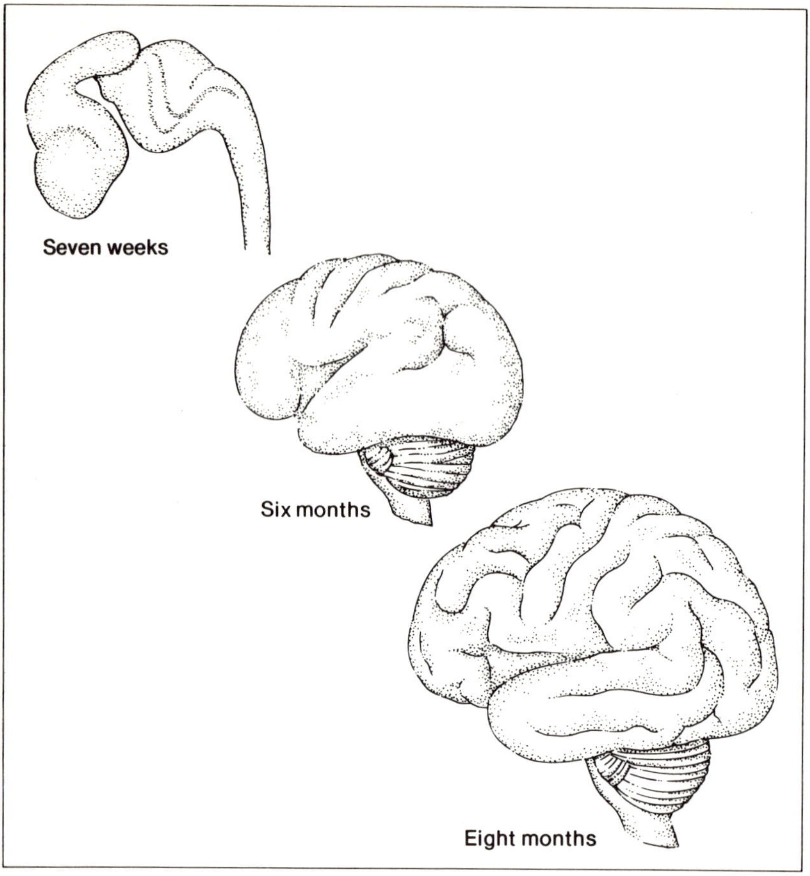

Figure 6. Stages of human brain development. At seven weeks, the brain can be seen as a still-continuous folding tube, expanding in the head region and with the cerebral lobes just beginning to form (clearly more mature than the rat embryo in Figure 5). At six months the cerebral lobes cover most of the rest of the brain, but their cortex has yet to expand to produce the characteristic folds seen at eight months and even more prominently in the newborn. ▶

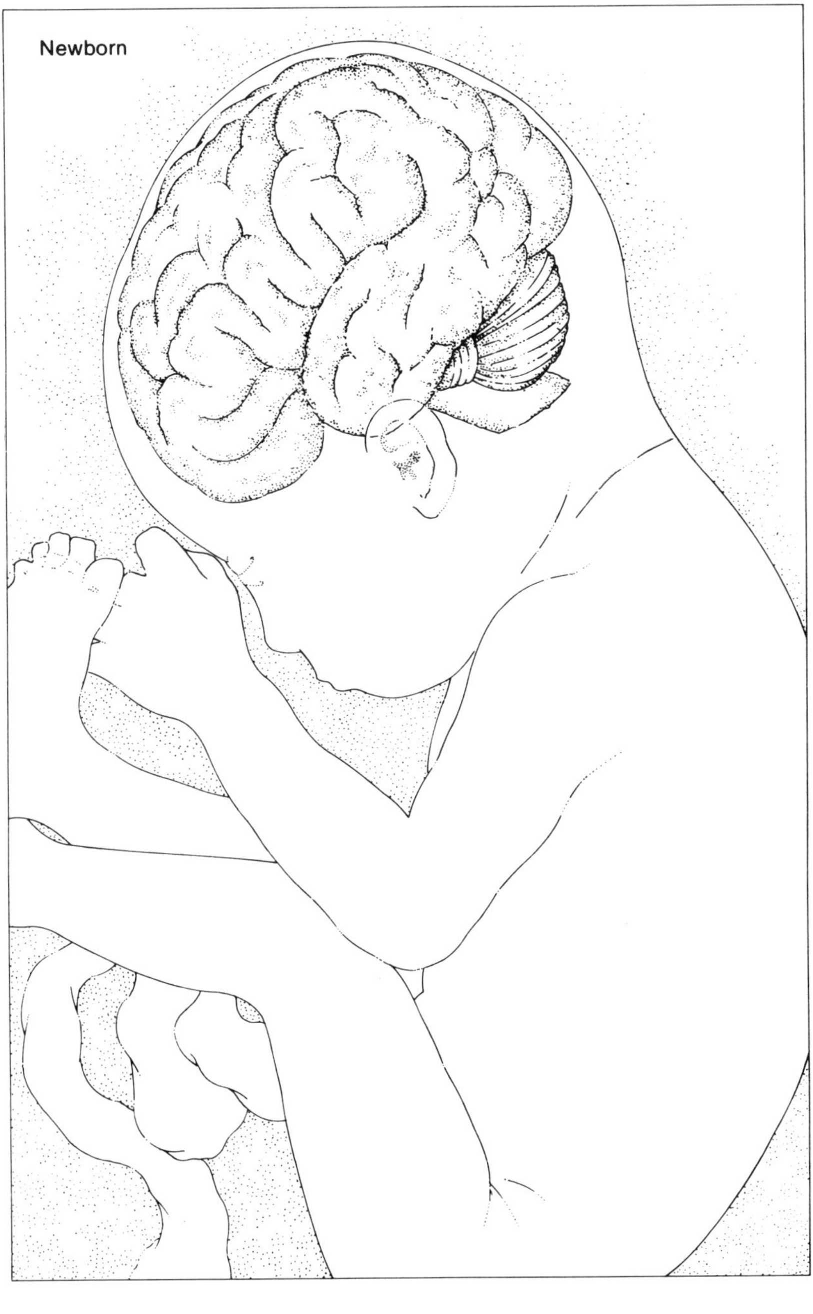
Newborn

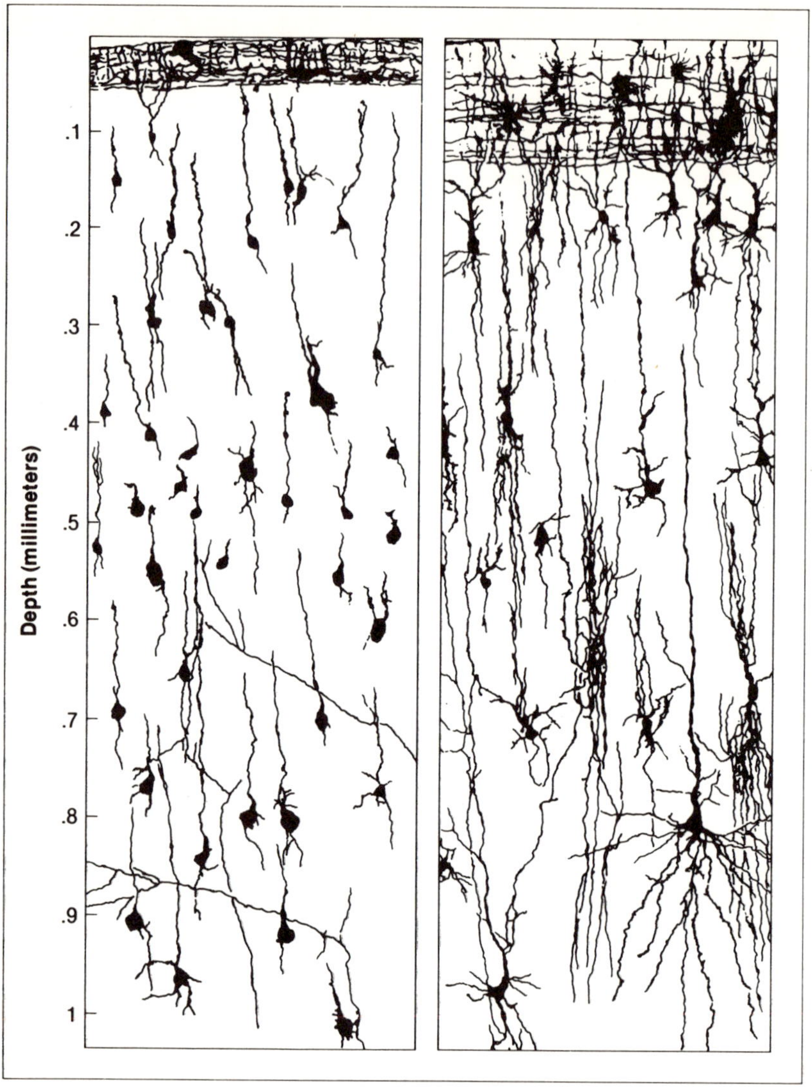

Figure 7. Neuronal maturation in the human cerebral cortex. The drawing to the left shows cell bodies and elongating processes at 25 weeks, that to the right at 33 weeks. In the intervening period the cortex has doubled in thickness. The other striking change is the increased number and length of processes and the increased complexity of interconnection. The "connectivity pattern" continues to become more complex during infancy and early childhood. After drawings kindly supplied by Dr. Dom Purpura, Albert Einstein Medical College.

degree of connection among them as important indices (38). Higher manifestations of self are clearly minimal before birth, but the possibility of gradual emergence of a rudiment of self, or of at least diffuse sentience, certainly cannot be excluded during the second and certainly the third trimester.

Fetal Infants

In this connection, observations on premature infants are relevant. Capability for survival, given adequate life support systems, reaches marginal levels by about 26 weeks of development. Gesell (39) has studied the behavior of such prematurely born "fetal-infants" at 28 to 32, 32 to 36, and 36 to 40 weeks, using cinematography to provide records for detailed analysis. His characterization of the 28- to 32-week stage is of a "loosely articulated mannikin" whose arms and legs are flaccid and whose head also is flaccidly attached to the neck and trunk. In the controlled environment of an incubator, if disturbed in any way, "he becomes briefly active but soon dissolves into a limp and torporous desuetude. This ever-recurring torpor is, in fact, his most conspicuous and consistent behavior . . . . There are no clear-cut distinctions to be made between activity and rest. Movements are meagre, fleeting and poorly sustained. Their terminations are more evident than their beginnings; he is always lapsing into inaction. But even this apparent lethargy lacks decisiveness. He is seldom completely quiescent for any length of time. The eyes may be open—or they may not. Or one eye may be open and the other closed. The lids may flutter. He seems to drowse when the eyes are open as well as when they are closed. Indeed, his state is so ambiguous that one scarcely knows whether he is still asleep when he moves or whether he may not actually be awake even when quiescent. His torpor is shallow and has little structure or temporal pattern. He is easily roused to brief mild activity, but he is never fully roused. He neither sleeps nor wakes, but only drowses and stirs."

The fetal infant of this stage makes mild response to light, sound, and mechanical stimuli. The responses, however, quickly peter out to "drowsy quiescence." Muscle tone is "minimal and fluctuating," seeming to increase and decrease locally in a wandering manner. The head and facial regions seem "to be alive, albeit not attentively alert." Many fragmented and uncoordinated facial gestures occur, enough so that "one might conclude that Nature is preparing the fetal infant for a histrionic career." This spasmodic and fractured gesturing clearly is premonitory to meaningful facial expressions of a later time.

The 32- to 36-week fetal infant is described as a midstage of maturation—more firmly integrated and, relatively speaking, more powerful. "Nonetheless, activity is more likely to occur as a reaction to handling or to any disturbance of his natural apathy." The stage is still "weak, indifferent and unresponsive." Moving objects do evoke some response, but without "inspectional regard" or fixation. The most important developmental advance is capacity for brief periods of wakeful alertness. "Out of this amorphous anlage, true wakefulness first begins to differentiate during the midstage of fetal-infancy. Again and again during the day (and night) he pricks the surface of mere being with moments of true wakefulness. The frank though as yet only occasional open-eyedness, the hunger cry even though feeble, the stirrings of discomfort are so many glimmers of wakefulness. Sleep, however, remains indecisive; he is, on the whole, an indisputably drowsy individual."

Gesell suggests that the fetal infant "is more than a mere spinal creature," that "the thalamic region (of the brain) is apparently sufficiently advanced to support a simple, undiscriminating type of awareness." The thalamic region is subcortical but part of the higher brain, in the adult connected to the cortex by an extensive radiation of nerve fibers. Gesell's suggestion is that the thalamus precedes the cortex in maturation and may be the site of a primitive awareness. He elaborates the notion: "even at the thalamic level, the infant's life is not limited to feeding and sleeping. While awake, he is also dimly aware. He begins to enjoy the exercise of his growing powers of awareness. This keeps him awake. So he awakes, not only for sheer necessity, but also for sensori-motor satisfactions." These impressionistic statements, based upon Gesell's long observation of infant and child behavior, imply that shortly before normal term, at 40 weeks, the rudiment of selfness, flickering and fluctuating, may be making its first appearance.

The Newborn and Beyond

Whatever the precise time of origin of the rudiment of self, its subsequent maturation is extended. The behavioral repertoire of the newborn is still an extremely limited basis on which to judge its degree of selfness. There is clear evidence of tactile, visual, auditory, and olfactory response, but, as noted by Munn (40), "we know nothing at all about the experiences, if any, which these stimuli and stimulus differences arouse." Not only can infants not tell us what they experience, but "our own early life is, experientially, a complete blank." Munn points out that malformed infants born without a brain have the usual repertoire of behavior and that brain injuries produced at birth do not affect behavior until months later. He concludes that "behavior during the prenatal period, and for some time after birth, thus appears to be controlled subcortically."

The judgment is in accord with what is known neurologically about cortical maturation. The various regions of the cortex mature at different times, but there is obvious continuing cortical maturation, both generalized and local, through infancy and on into childhood. For example, Tanner (41) notes that during the first two years after birth the most mature part of the cortex is the primary motor area whose neurones project to and initiate action in muscles all over the body. The primary sensory area is less advanced, still less is the primary visual area, and least advanced among the sensory areas is the auditory area. During this time the associational areas—communicators and integrators of sensory and motor inputs and outputs—are fairly uniformly in a lesser maturational state than the sensory and motor areas themselves.

Within each primary area there are similar differences in level of maturation. In the motor area the subregions producing movement of the arms and trunk are further developed than those producing movements of the legs. The leg areas remain poorly developed until near the end of the second year. All of these maturational changes, as seen at the cellular level, accord well with the changing behavior of the developing child.

Recently, much attention has been given to still more detailed correlations between structural and functional maturation of higher brain centers in both animals and humans. On the one hand, optical and electron microscopic observations are revealing new facts about the multiplicity and the complexities of the connections among the cortical nerve cells. On the other hand, increasingly sophisticated techniques allow detection of patterns of electrical activity accompanying nerve cell activity that underlies behavior. Combining these two, it is clear, for example, that advancing complexity of connections among cortical nerve cells correlates closely with advancing maturation recorded by electroencephalography (42). Levels of detectable connections among nerve cells in certain brain regions thus become a crude measure of probable function in those regions. It is striking that in the newborn animal, when cortical maturation is still early, nerve cell maturation in the subcortical reticular formation is essentially complete. The reticular formation is necessary for integration of such vital internal processes as respiration and heartbeat and for primitive, reflexive behaviors such as sucking, swallowing, early vocalization, and generalized limb movements. These behaviors therefore may be interpreted as supraspinal but subcortical.

Continuous Genesis of Self

What is suggested by this accumulating evidence is that self does not arise at a given moment but rather is the product of processes of continuing genesis, beginning *in utero* but continuing well after birth. Self almost certainly is not actually present during the first two months of development, although it becomes increasingly imminent. In these terms the period of reasonable certainty that no semblance of self exists ends with the appearance of spontaneous and responsive behavior. Beyond this point scientific judgment must be progressively more qualified, depending upon what assumptions are made.

If the assumption is that all spontaneous and responsive behavior involves a degree of sentience that represents a minimal manifestation of self, then the developing human becomes such a minimal self at roughly eight weeks. The assumption, however, would admit most animals and, depending upon the detail of definition, possibly all life to the category of selfhood.

If the assumption is added that the spontaneous and responsive behavior must be based upon sensorimotor reflex chains of nerve cells including a central nervous system, then in addition to the developing human at eight weeks, higher animals, including insects, are admitted to the category of selfness. This can be avoided, of course, by arbitrarily limiting consideration to the human species.

If a further assumption is made that the sensorimotor reflexes must involve at least the reticular formation in the human brain, then current evidence suggests that selfness may not arise until at least the beginning of the third trimester, in approximate relation to onset of capability for independent respiration. Under this assumption the earliest fetal infants that can survive without artificial respiratory support would be admitted to selfhood. This is the point when the fetus is usually said to be "viable," given the current status of life support technology for premature infants.

Finally, if the existence of self is assumed to be inextricably tied to some level of cortical influence on behavior, then even the newborn may not yet have attained selfhood. As indicated above, the evidence is equivocal as to whether the behavioral repertoire of the newborn is cortically dependent. The level of cortical maturation in the newborn is, although not uniform over its entire extent, generally quite immature.

The Human Recognition Factor

These assumptions focus on biological criteria of selfness as they bear upon a minimal experiential state of bounded sentience. What has just been said about assumptions in defining a stage of minimal self-status also emphasizes that the definition is highly sensitive to judgmental factors. The scientific information is determinative only in that it excludes any significant level of sentience during approximately the first eight weeks of human development. Beyond that point suitable assumptions can include or exclude significant sentience right up to birth itself. Given this circumstance, the third criterion of recognition of self by others potentially is of major importance.

As a first approximation, the rationale of the criterion rests on the established expectation that other people have inner selves like our own. That being the case, the question is to determine when in development the embryo or fetus is generally recognizable as human and evokes empathy as another self. Prior to that point, assumption of the presence of an inner self requires some objective evidence of its existence. Subsequent to that point, the burden of proof shifts. A self is to be assumed unless there is strong evidence to the contrary. The question thus becomes the stage at which the embryo or fetus can first be generally recognized as human, generating empathy as a person or a person-to-be.

Examination of human embryos (Figure 8) shows that structural characteristics recognizably human to a lay person are present at least by twelve to thirteen weeks of development. This is at the end of the first trimester, the time at which it has been traditional to change the term embryo to fetus as the designation for the developing human. Although the fetus at this stage has a lot of developing to do and is by no means a miniature person needing simply to be scaled up by growth, a number of critical features for recognition are present. The head is disproportionately large and the legs are tiny, but the general body configuration is recognizably human. In contrast to earlier stages, a definite face is present, a critical characteristic for human recognition. Also, hands and feet, including fingers and toes, are well defined and unquestionably human. It is also important to note that responsive movements at this stage are quite strong and that spontaneous movement is beginning. Although the fetus is still very small, almost any observer is likely to regard it as human and at least a person-to-be.

Whether a given observer will assume the presence of a self and exhibit empathy is a more difficult question on which there appear to be few data. It is at this point that the criterion becomes difficult to deal with in practical terms. Professionals accustomed to dealing with abortuses might be expected to react differently from lay people. Sex, age, and cultural differences might be expected. Even the context in which the fetus is being viewed might be expected to affect reactions. Certainly the degree to which the fetus not only looked human but behaved in human ways would have considerable impact.

The important point to be made in the present discussion is that human recognition would not suggest the probable presence of self-status *any earlier* than the end of the first trimester. It would, however, become a progressively more significant factor beyond that point as both appearance and behavior of the fetus mature. So far as external fertilization is concerned, application of the human recognition criterion would suggest that, unless strong evidence for its existence were presented, an inner self would not be expected to be present at the early stages that are currently exteriorized and manipulated. With respect to abortion, the situation would reverse at the beginning of the second trimester. More and more people might assume the presence of some level of self, and evidence to the contrary would need to be stronger and stronger to persuade them otherwise. This is the developmental interval where value judgments are crucial and the political process must be effective. At the moment policy in the United States as it refers to abortion is based upon an uneasy consensus and continuing controversy. It is likely to be a long time (if ever) before the matter of self-states in later development can be resolved by decisive scientific information. From the information presented in this chapter, however, the existence of self-states at stages involved in external human fertilization appears quite unlikely.

Figure 8. Human embryos of about 6, 7, 8, and 13 weeks of development. The 6-week stage is still rudimentary in almost all respects, the 7-week stage is maturing but still not obviously human, the 8-week has "humanoid" limbs, and the 13-week stage probably would be recognized by most observers as an immature infant (fetus). After photographs kindly supplied by the Department of Embryology (Davis), Carnegie Institution of Washington. ▶

Human Embryos

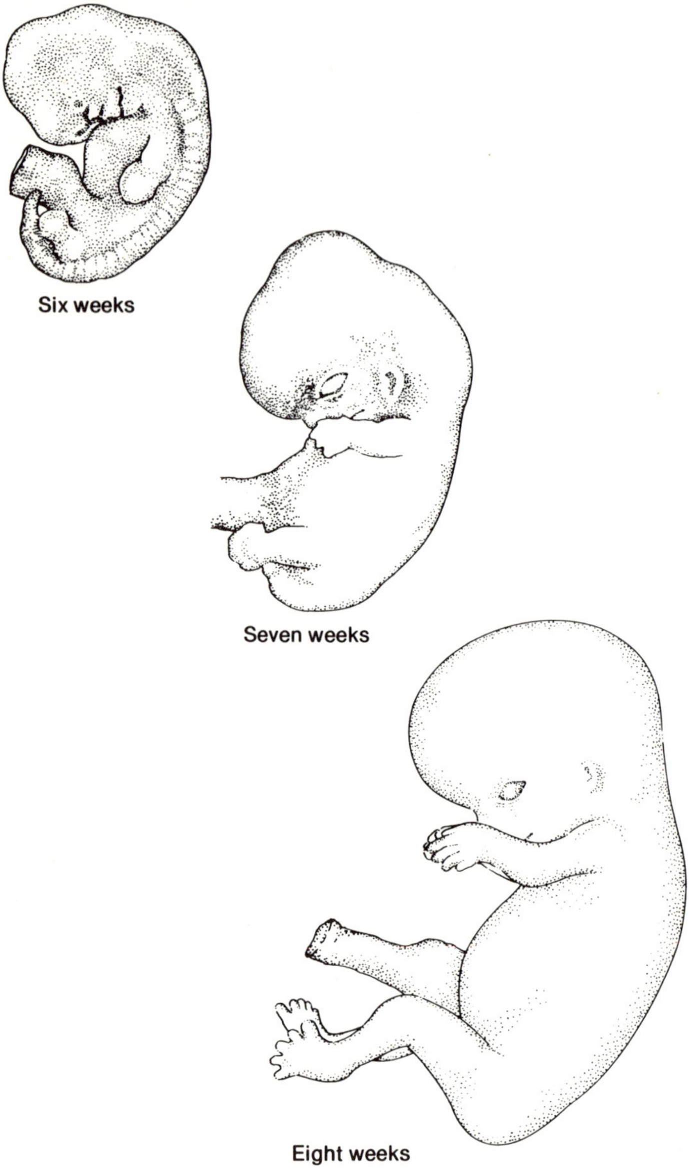

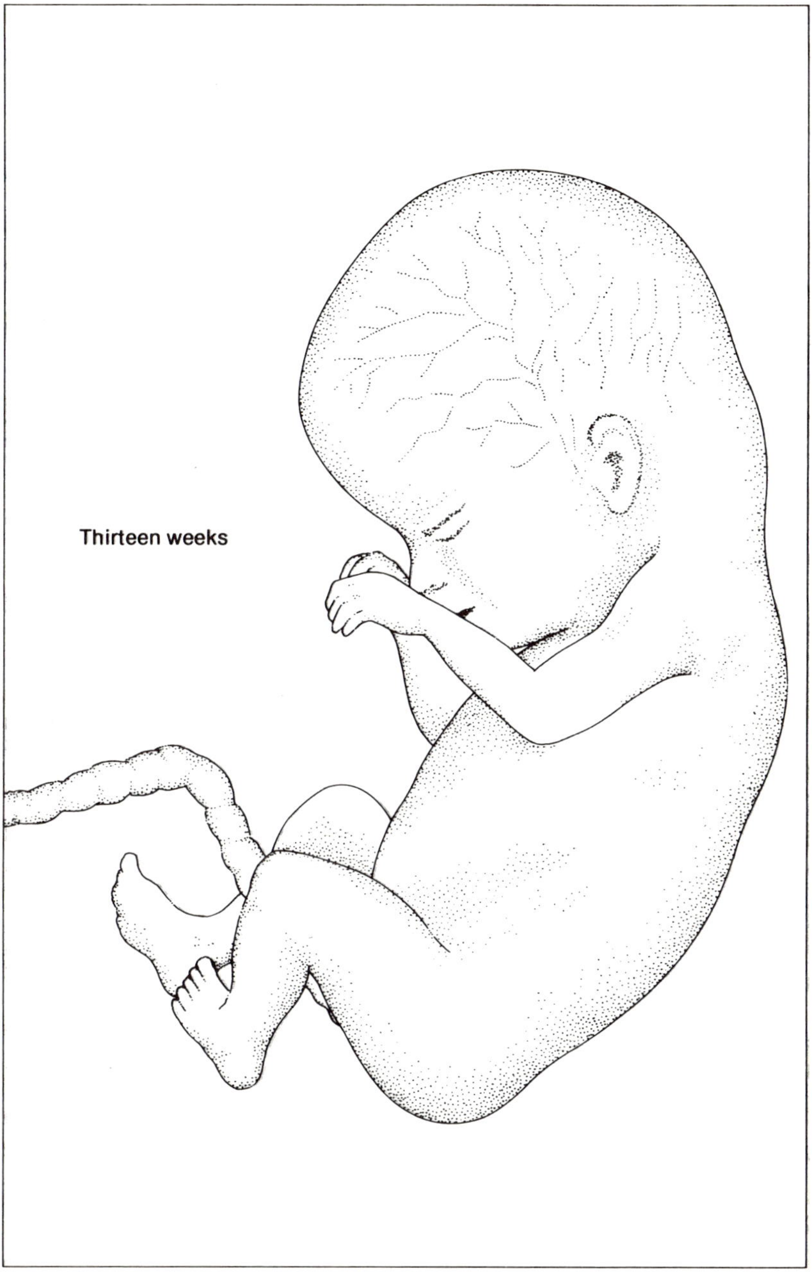

Thirteen weeks

GENERAL REFERENCES

Edelman, G. M., and Mountcastle, V. B., *The Mindful Brain*. Cambridge: MIT Press (1978).

Gallup, G. G., Self-awareness in primates. *Amer. Sci.* 67: 417–421 (1979).

Gesell, A., *The Embryology of Human Behavior.* Westport, Connecticut: Greenwood Press (1971).

Globus, M. G., and Savodnik, I. (eds.), *Consciousness and the Brain. A Scientific and Philosophical Inquiry.* New York: Plenum (1976).

Humphrey, T., Function of the nervous system during prenatal life. In U. Stave (ed.), *Perinatal Physiology,* Chapter 30. New York: Plenum (1978).

Moore, R. Y., The developmental organization of the fetal brain. In L. Gluck, (ed.), *Intrauterine Asphyxia and the Developing Fetal Brain*. Chicago: Year Book Medical Publishers (1977).

Munn, N. L., *The Evolution and Growth of Human Behavior*. Boston: Houghton Mifflin (1974).

Popper, K. R., and Eccles, J. C., *The Self and Its Brain*. Springer (1977).

Tanner, J. M., *Foetus into Man.* Cambridge, Mass.: Harvard Univ. Press (1978).

Uttal, W. R., *The Psychobiology of Mind.* Hillsdale, N.J.: Lawrence Erlbaum Associates, Distributed by Halsted Press, Division of J. Wiley (1978).

Chapter VI

Looking Ahead—Options and Decisions

With the advent of external human fertilization we have reached a new high ground of potential options with respect to our own reproduction. How much of the potential we should utilize and what options we should exercise will very likely be debated for decades and possibly for generations to come. For some, such new heights are exhilarating, for others they are fearsome. For all, they offer a new perspective, a moment to look back down the trail to familiar terrain and ahead to a misty future. In theory we might choose to turn back, but in reality the overall thrust of all life and certainly of human life is onward and upward. Life rarely goes home again.

Where do we stand, and what is the view ahead? We have outlined our present location in previous chapters. Clearly we face a number of options, both near and long-term. Clearly, also, there are differences of opinion as to the next best steps. How do we now assess our position and achieve at least operational consensus on a future course? That is the subject of this chapter.

The process of assessment has barely begun. It is one for which we have no ample precedent. It is true that in recent years the rapid pace of technological advance has spawned a new analytical thrust known as technology assessment. Its objective is to apply rational analysis and forecasting to policy decision-making with respect to new technologies, especially to the promises and problems they present. The objective is laudable and the general philosophy appropriate. It has not, however, yet been demonstrated that there are methodologies or formulas for decision-making that can substitute for hard cogitation, considerable controversy, and the exercise of sound judgment. Especially is this true when we confront not a single technological advance but a broad front of considerable breadth and depth.

A first effort along these general lines was made by the HEW Ethics Advisory Board appointed by then-Secretary Joseph Califano in September, 1977. The Board had before it a specific research application for support of risk assessment research bearing on external human fertilization. The application was referred for ethical evaluation, but the Board was especially charged by the Secretary to examine very broadly the issues raised because of the recent first birth resulting from external human fertilization. Secretary Califano sent a special communication to the first meeting of the Board containing its special charge (see Appendix I). He asked the Board to conduct a wide-ranging inquiry of the scientific, ethical, legal, and social issues involved in the general procedure, with as much public participation as possible. Essentially, the Secretary sought the equivalent of a national debate on the subject to give guidance to official decision-making.

The Board consisted of fifteen members and had eight staff assistants. The chairman was James C. Gaither, a distinguished San Francisco attorney. The vice-chairman was David A. Hamburg, an equally distinguished psychiatrist and President of the Institute of Medicine. Other members included six physicians, one the Dean of the Harvard Medical School and another the Dean of the School of Hygiene and Public Health at Johns Hopkins University. Two members were experts in medical ethics, and three were lay persons biomedically but distinguished in public affairs. Two of the fifteen members were women. Overall, the Board might be judged weighty in authority and expertise yet not fully representative of the United States population nor of the complex interests involved. However, its report (Appendix II) represents an important step in formulating sound public policy in this difficult, consequential, and controversial area.

The Calculus of Benefit, Risk, and Social Worth

A prominent issue before the Board was the probable benefit to be gained by clinical use of external human fertilization, in relation to imaginable risks and possible options.

Estimating the benefit starts simply enough. What could be clearer and stronger than the benefit to a sterile couple of obtaining their own child? There is no doubt about the intensity of motivation of many such couples. They will travel long distances for medical advice, they will bear high costs often beyond their means, and they will accept almost any reasonable risk to satisfy their desire. For a child-hungry sterile couple, external fertilization offers a means to meet a deeply felt need.

Moreover, the Board reported wide public support for use of the new technology. A Gallup poll taken in August, 1978, shortly after the announcement of the first such birth in England, showed that 53% of the sample would themselves resort to the procedure if they were married and could not have a child, 36% said they would not do so, and the rest were undecided. An even higher fraction among those between 18 and 30 years old—two-thirds—said that they would agree to the procedure if they required it. This group is, of course, the one most likely to have children in the next decade. Further, 60% of the sampled group favored availability of the procedure to anyone who needed and wanted it. In none of these responses was there significant difference between men and women. A Harris poll taken at about the same time gave essentially similar results.

There is, therefore, a strong publicly perceived attractiveness to the new reproductive technology when it is applied to alleviate sterility. The public response, incidentally, appeared to be an informed one. The Gallup poll found that "an extraordinary 93% had heard or read about the baby," and 42% were able to give a full and correct explanation of the procedure. Is this enough to conclude that the procedure yields a net benefit? For the individuals to be directly benefited, probably yes, but not necessarily for society as a whole. Experience with dialysis machines for kidney disease, for example, have made many people ask further questions about new medical technologies. How many people will be benefited by the new procedure, will various subpopulations benefit approximately equally, what are likely to be the costs relative to the benefits, and how will the costs be covered?

Sterility due to blockage of oviducts has been estimated roughly to occur in perhaps 500,000 American women. Only some fraction of these would be in child-bearing years and hence candidates for external fertilization at a given time. Let us assume that of all women with obstructed oviducts, one-fourth are of child-bearing age (18 to 35 years old) and that two-thirds who fit the category will actually seek the procedure (as suggested by the data of the Gallup poll). On the basis of these crude assumptions, approximately 100,000 American women might want the procedure. If we assume a cost of $5000 per case (a clinic recently authorized in Virginia is preliminarily estimating $4000) (43), the total cost for all of these women to have one child would be almost $0.5 billion. If we assume that 10% might seek the procedure in a given year, the annual cost would be about $50 million.

Critics of the procedure, looking at comparable rough estimates, have voiced concern and reservation about its worth as an overall *social* benefit. Some charge that external fertilization represents misallocation of both effort and funds that might be better spent for other, more basic, health benefits. They regard the procedure as an example of expensive, high-technology medicine, aimed at the needs of relatively few couples in higher income strata and unlikely to be available to low-income couples, who would require subsidy. Current legislation restricting public funding of abortion is cited as evidence of the financial bind.

Critics further suggest that, with respect to the problem of sterility, preventive measures are more likely than technological therapy to produce favorable long-term effects—and at lower social costs. For example, a major cause of obstruction of the oviducts is pelvic inflammation, especially incident to gonorrhea. Greater emphasis on sexual hygiene could significantly reduce the need for technological intervention. Moreover, it is argued that, although surgical repair of the oviduct is difficult and therefore successful in only a minority of cases, its effectiveness might be improved by greater investment in research in that direction. Note is taken, also, of adoption as a way to meet the needs of sterile couples, since, in many instances, genetic relationship does not seem essential for a satisfying parental role. Some critics, who are also critics of the health care system in the United States in general, allege that the benefit of gaining a child via external fertilization is at the cost of further subjugation of both mother and child to a system that is steadily becoming more remote through excessive professionalization and specialization. In consequence, as in this instance, treatment is more and more complex and sophisticated but less and less comprehensible and controllable by the patient.

What begins, therefore, as a simple and clear-cut benefit for a particular couple becomes far more complex and debatable at the social level. This is especially the case when the *nature of the procedure* is taken into account, for the procedure, as noted in Chapter IV, clearly impacts on a set of fundamental social values that currently are in transition and widely debated.

Ethics Review Board Conclusions

In recognition of these complexities, the Ethics Advisory Board's conclusions (see Appendix II) are cautious, dealing as much as possible with immediately presented matters and avoiding commitment with respect to most others. A potential benefit for women afflicted by infertility is accepted, but with reservations. Conceding that the procedure may be "for some women . . . the only way to bear children of their own," the Board notes the limitation that it does not yet appear to be "very effective . . . a number of attempts have been necessary before a pregnancy in a particular woman can be established, if at all." It also notes that "many questions remain as to the safety of the procedure for the offspring."

Nonetheless, the Board realistically foresees that "clinics may soon be established, both in this country and abroad," to make the technique available to infertile couples. Given this reality, the Board's recommendations amount to an admonition to proceed with caution. Thus, "The Board is concerned about still unanswered questions of safety . . . about the physical and mental health of the children born . . . and about their legal status." However, "Many women have told the Board that in order to bear a child of their own they will submit to whatever risks are involved. The Board believes that while the Department should not interfere with such reproductive decisions, it has a legitimate interest in developing and disseminating information regarding safety and health so that fully informed choices about reproduction can be made."

The Board goes further, however, than suggesting a purely informational federal role. Its first formal conclusion is a recommendation for support of research on animals to obtain better understanding, to assess risks, and to improve efficacy of the procedure. "Careful research with animal models might provide a more accurate estimate of the chances of achieving a successful pregnancy. It might also reduce the inconvenience and risk to women of undergoing multiple procedures to establish a pregnancy by improving techniques for recovering ova, identifying embryonic abnormalities and achieving implantation."

The Board's second formal conclusion finds research directly on humans in relation to external fertilization ethically acceptable with certain provisos. First, the Board distinguishes between what is "clearly ethically right" and what is "ethically defensible but still legitimately controverted." The Board's conclusions are specified as relating to the second ethical standpoint; the Board emphasizes "that it is *not* finding that the ethical considerations against such research are insubstantial." The following stipulations are then added: If the research does not involve transfer of embryos back to the uterus, it must nonetheless comply with regulations governing research with human subjects; it must be *primarily directed* toward safety and efficacy of transfer of embryos back to the uterus, yielding information not available through other means; donors of eggs and sperm must be afforded fully informed consent; no embryos should be carried beyond the stage of implantation; public announcement must be made as soon as any evidence develops of higher rates of embryonic abnormality than in natural human reproduction; and, in the event of transfer of embryos, it "should be attempted only with gametes obtained from lawfully married couples."

The Board's third formal conclusion extends *ethical* sanction to *federal support* of human research, subject to the same stipulations outlined in the second conclusion. It specifically does *not*, however, "address the question of the level of funding, if any, which such research might be given." Noting the complexity of the issues involved in relation to the kind and degree of federal support, the Board "defers to established political, scientific and administrative procedures for allocating public research funds." This decision is justified by the belief that funding decisions "should be made in the larger context where all relevant data and arguments—scientific, political, economic, legal and ethical—can be considered."

The Board further notes that potentially valuable knowledge might result from research on human embryos without transfer to the uterus, knowledge unrelated to alleviation of sterility. "The Board makes no judgment at this time regarding the ethical acceptability of such research nor does it speculate about what research might be sufficiently compelling to justify the use of human embryos." It is noted that "concerns regarding the moral status of the embryo and the potential long-range consequences of this research were among the most difficult that confronted the Board." Agreement was reached that "the human embryo is entitled to profound respect; but this respect does not necessarily encompass the full legal and moral rights attributed to persons." Accordingly, the Board asked that any applications for support of research of this kind be submitted to it for review.

The report of the Board containing these and several other conclusions was forwarded to the Secretary of Health and Human Services (formerly Health, Education and Welfare) on May 4, 1979, and on June 19, 1979, it was published in the Federal Register. More than a year later, having received 13,000 public comments that are said informally to have been mainly adverse, the Secretary had taken no action. Meanwhile, Congress had created a President's Commission for the Study of Ethical Problems in Medicine and Biomedical and Behavioral Research, a successor to the National Commission for the Protection of Human Subjects. The Ethics Advisory Board was terminated shortly thereafter, ostensibly because the new Commission's charge overlapped that of the Board.

On February 21, 1980, Senators Edward Kennedy and Orin Hatch had requested that the new Commission review and comment on the Ethics Advisory Board's report. In a letter of May 21, 1980, Commission Chairman Morris B. Abram reported to Senator Kennedy that the Commissioners had complied with the request and "were satisfied by the adequacy and thoroughness of the procedures used," that "the conclusions of the Board seem well supported," and that "the Commission may take up additional issues in the future." The Chairman made clear, however, that "the Commission does not pass judgment one way or the other on the merits of any specific conclusion." The Chairman further noted that the Commission's own charge might require it to examine additional aspects of the matter of external fertilization but that it did not wish its efforts to be "premature or duplicative" pending a conclusion by the Secretary of Health and Human Resources on the report of the Ethics Advisory Board. One cannot help but remark that the Commission recognized a hot potato when it saw one. Nonetheless, federal policy remains unclear until either the Secretary or the President's Commission takes some action.

External Human Fertilization in Clinical Operation

Successful cases of external human fertilization have now been reported from England, India, and Australia. These "firsts" stemmed from groups that had been involved for some time in background research. Several clinical groups at medical schools began preparations to test or use the technique shortly after its success was announced. The first group in the United States to move formally to make the technique widely available is located at the Norfolk General Hospital. This group received clearance from the State of Virginia to proceed with necessary facilities modification on January 25, 1980. The clearance was in the form of a certificate of need allowing the hospital to renovate space for the Norfolk Clinic, a center for treatment of infertility. Virginia's health commissioner, in giving his approval (reported in the press on January 9), said that, after five months of hearings and studies, it was determined that the proposed facility would violate no state or federal law. The project was also "blessed" by the Committee on Human Experimentation and Research of Eastern Virginia Medical School, after what was described as the most careful scrutiny ever given by this Committee to a submitted treatment plan.

The proposal received neither approval nor blessing from the Tidewater chapter of the Virginia Society for Human Life. Its president said that he would appeal the decision immediately. He was quoted further: "We'll never give up. There's a lot of pressure against it. And a lot more is mounting. This isn't the end of it." Clearly, the possibility exists that the courts will again be asked to rule on issues raised by opponents of a significant new technology.

Meanwhile the Norfolk Clinic has been moving ahead, not only with technological preparation but with the design of medical criteria for appropriate patient selection and other aspects of sound medical practice (43). Among the selection criteria adopted are the following: (1) an otherwise healthy, childless, married couple; (2) a stable marriage, as clinically determined; (3) no known alternative to achieve pregnancy; (4) age of wife between 25 and 35; (5) ability to pay an estimated cost of $4000 (not covered by most medical insurance programs and specifically excluded by Blue Cross in Virginia). By March, 1980, "a significant number of couples from among thousands inquiring" were reported to have been selected and to be undergoing treatment at the Clinic.

Because the Norfolk Clinic is a general fertility cinic, it is interested in using other procedures than external fertilizaion to treat blocked oviducts. Reportedly it is attempting transfer of unfertilized eggs into the uterus of the donor, both subsequent and prior to natural intercourse with the husband. This is an attempt to eliminate an external phase by obtaining fertilization directly in the uterus. There also is interest in using the external procedure to alleviate male infertility. The sperm count required for success of the external process is lower than that for natural intercourse (or for artificial insemination, which requires a still higher count). A subminimal ejaculate for normal fertilization might be entirely adequate for the laboratory-assisted process. The philosophy of the Clinic, therefore, is to incorporate external fertilization into the armamentarium of standard medical practice as applied to infertility. It is expected by the Clinic that many both anticipated and unanticipated problems will arise in the process.

Some of these problems are likely to stem from the social context within which the new technique is being initiated. Limitation of its use to married couples fits established traditional mores but almost certainly will be challenged by several nontraditional attitudes. Sterile women who choose to be single but do not wish to be childless may claim equal right to benefit from the technique. In justification of their claim, they can point to the large number of single-parent families resulting from divorce, as well as to the number of babies born out of wedlock. Similarly, limitation to married couples may be challenged by other women who, for economic or other reasons, do not wish or cannot go through pregnancy but nonetheless want a genetically related child. A probably feasible technical solution is insertion of the fertilized egg, whatever the genetic parentage, into the uterus of a psychologically and physiologically receptive surrogate who will carry it to term and then turn it over to the planned parent. Precedents for this have been reported in connection with artificial insemination (6). These variations of the basic procedure for external human fertilization are small technically but large in the social, ethical, and legal issues and problems they generate. Decisions about them must be regarded as belonging on the current public policy agenda. The preliminary policy adopted by the Norfolk Clinic is in accord with the Ethics Advisory Board's recommendation to the DHEW (now DHHS) Secretary, but, even if accepted, this recommendation carries no legal force beyond the Department's own activities. The Norfolk Clinic could change its policy at any time, and other facilities that may be established can adopt other policies. The question posed is whether there should be uniform and general *public* policy on the matter and, if so, how that policy should be established and what its content should be. The question involves value judgments, and its answer therefore must come out of a political process. This aspect will be taken up later in this chapter.

Where Might We Go?

Another important question on the public policy agenda is whether and how the now open window on early stages of human development should be exploited to gain new knowledge. The question can be viewed in two time-frames—relatively short-term (roughly a decade) and long-term. Central to both is the following issue: To what extent and under what circumstances should human eggs and early embryos be open to systematic observation and deliberate manipulation? All long-term options depend upon how this question is answered since observation and manipulation will be required to test each option. Consideration of this question therefore has short-term priority.

What are the policy options? A general prohibition of external human fertilization would formally close the window. United States citizens would then have to go abroad for this treatment of infertility, if we assume that not all countries would adopt the restrictive policy. This was the case some years ago for abortion. The procedure might be available covertly in the United States, under dubious professional standards, as was also the case with abortion. Whatever the social consequences, however, such a prohibition would eliminate for the moment, within the United States, the possible study of human eggs and early embryos. There is little evidence in public reactions to date that the course of prohibition will be embarked upon. There is, likewise, little evidence that federal funding for such research will be made available.

A second option is to allow or encourage only observations and manipulations intended directly to improve the safety and efficacy of the clinical procedure for external fertilization. This, in the main, was the recommendation of the Ethics Advisory Board. This option would allow some new experience and knowledge to be gained but only as a direct result or incidental by-product of the clinical objective. Little other knowledge or practical benefit could be deliberately sought.

A third option would be to allow or encourage observation and manipulations intended directly to serve other *specified purposes,* whether these be to gain knowledge or to serve practical ends. This would amount to controlled licensure, requiring a mechanism to define such purposes and to ensure compliance. It would acknowledge the special status of human eggs and embryos, protecting them from casual or inconsequential exploitation. At the same time, it would concede that they are not yet persons in any objective sense and that their use is legitimate when serious and socially accepted human purposes require it. The Ethics Advisory Board seems to have leaned slightly in this direction when it came to no conclusion "about what [other] research might be sufficiently compelling to justify the use of human embryos" but noted that existing DHEW regulations would require that "applications for support of such research should be submitted to the Board for ethical review." (However, the demise of the Board has essentially rendered this recommendation moot, recreating a *de facto* moratorium that existed before the Board was appointed. A possible way to remedy this would be to assign the responsibility to the current Institutional Review Boards. There are, however, procedural, logical, and philosophical reservations to such a course.)

A final option would be to define a stage in human development prior to which no protectable human entity exists, allowing scientific observation and manipulation to proceed as freely in these nonprotected stages as currently is done with human cells and tissues. Defining such a stage precisely has grave difficulties and also would neglect the special property of eggs and early embryos that allows them, under appropriate circumstances, to *become* a protectable person.

It is important to point out that the choice among the options can be considered in two contexts: (1) what is to be countenanced under any circumstance, and (2) what is to be encouraged and supported by the federal (or other) government. Given the current dominant federal role in the funding of biomedical research, the difference may not appear great. However, there is an important policy distinction philosophically that could become practically significant as well if, as many people believe to be desirable, support of research returned to a greater pluralism.

A Logistical Problem

Central to choice among these options is definition of the social and legal status of the early human embryo. In connection with the issue of abortion, an emotional, ethical debate has been raging that has created a smoke screen around the entire matter. The scientific considerations that bear upon it have been outlined in some detail in Chapter V. They indicate strongly that objective evidence provides no basis for assumption of even a semblance of a sentient self prior to about the eighth week of pregnancy. Preimplantation stages, based upon scientific observation, are essentially cellular. The process of becoming a supercellular entity is in only the earliest and still unstable stages. This scientific perception, however, is not likely to become the sole, or even dominant, determinant of policy in the immediate future. If it were, some variant of the fourth option might be adopted. Since it is not, the political equation makes something in the range of options two and three most reasonable. This is where the Ethics Advisory Board consensus came to rest.

How much difference is there between options two and three? Both accept *purpose* as a justification for invading what clearly is a gray zone in terms of the rights of personhood. Option two accepts only a single purpose as adequate justification—to provide a safe and efficacious procedure to alleviate infertility. Option three admits other purposes yet to be specified but presumably of comparable import and social acceptability to that accepted under option two. In the long run the difference is likely to be quite significant; in the short run the significance is unlikely to be great. This is because a major limitation on successful research using human eggs and early embryos is logistical.

Even if much time and trouble is expended by both investigator and volunteer subjects, it is virtually impossible to get a satisfactory supply of human eggs and early embryos for effective scientific investigation or even definitive clinical trials. Barring the use of hormones to induce superovulation (at the moment to be avoided because of possible effects on both the egg and the donor), at best only one egg per donor per month might be obtained—perhaps a hundred eggs per year from ten donors! Moreover, the eggs are tiny, severely limiting biochemical study. Supply might be augmented by use of ovaries surgically removed for other reasons, but this source is irregular and variable in ways that affect experimental quality. Therefore, even without ethical, social, and economic barriers, the human female is a poor "experimental animal" for studies of early embryos. At the present stage of understanding the mouse is very much to be preferred, although even it does not match the frog, chicken, or sea urchin in experimental advantage.

If and when it becomes critically important to work with human eggs and early embryos—and it seems likely that it eventually will—the logistical problem will have to be solved. No reasonable person would contemplate a solution based on human "egg-layers," whether volunteer or paid. There is, however, an imaginable alternative whose feasibility is yet to be demonstrated. Testing of this alternative would best be done on the mouse, where, for other purposes, some steps already have been taken and where the whole process would have logistical advantages as well. It would include external fertilization, external development of the embryo to the stage of early formation of the ovary, organ culture of the rudiments of the ovary to produce mature eggs, and use of the eggs for external fertilization to initiate a new cycle. Knowledge necessary to complete such a cycle in mice would require the following: (1) improvement of techniques for ectogenesis to carry mouse embryos from external fertilization to stages of organogenesis such as have been accomplished in the rat; and (2) improved techniques for developing rudimentary ovaries to yield mature eggs in organ culture. Neither of these steps appears insurmountable technically if given sufficient attention. The result would be the capability to turn over generations of mice in culture without ever producing adults. This could shorten mouse generation times from several months to several weeks. In addition to its logistical advantages, combination of this technique with embryo fusion, nuclear transplantation, and diploidization should yield new opportunities for more refined genetic and developmental analyses in mice.

Were the procedure successful in mice, it probably could eventually be applied, considering the question of technical feasibility alone, to the human species. Since it would yield an increased number of eggs (sperm not being a problem) and would not involve development beyond early organogenesis in any generation, it could both solve the logistical problem and reduce the ethical problem. The latter would occur if and when a consensus was reached to exclude from protection as a person, or to license for use for accepted purposes, human developmental stages prior to stages of brain maturation judged necessary for simple sentience. It would then be possible to test, *within agreed human purpose,* knowledge gained about early stages of the mouse on similar human stages under comparable circumstances. Insertion of such embryos into a uterus for continued development would, of course, not be intended or sanctioned without a separate and further intensive scientific, medical, ethical, and public scrutiny to ensure that it served essential and established human purposes and met the highest ethical criteria.

Some such procedure, whether of this or other kind, would be necessary to provide an adequate number of human eggs and early embryos for any sanctioned successful experimentation. Unless such a procedure becomes available, there is little practical difference between options two and three in what we would currently define as a short-term prospect. The necessary foundation for any direct experimental approaches to early human development must first be built in studies of the mouse (or other suitable small species with relatively short generation time). Meanwhile, also, growing experience in handling early human embryos to deal with sterility problems may lessen anxiety and give opportunity for calm examination and sound decisions about future options.

Rationales for Intervention

What rationales are there for even considering future wider interventions in early human development? In general terms, the rationale is to utilize expanding options and capability to make beneficial choices in terms of purpose rather than of accident or chance. As a specific example, consider an obvious dichotomy based upon chance—the determination of sex type. As is well known, sex type normally is *genetically* established at fertilization, based upon a visibly dissimilar pair of chromosomes known as X and Y. These are unusual in their *visible* dissimilarity but not at all unusual in exerting dissimilar genetic effects. Dissimilarities exist, in fact, in each chromosomal pair, since the two members are from different parents. In the case of human sex-determining chromosomes, if an offspring receives a pair that is visibly similar—that is, XX—the offspring is genetically female; if the pair is visibly dissimilar—XY—the offspring is genetically male. The differential depends upon the fact that males produce two kinds of sperm in equal quantity, X-bearing and Y-bearing. The genetic sex of the offspring is determined at fertilization by the chance event of one or the other kind of sperm. In very general terms the chances are fifty-fifty, a not unimportant ratio biologically and socially.

As is also well-known, many people care about which sex their offspring will be. Some prefer one sex, some the other, and some would like both but in a particular sequence. Various schemes have been proposed to control the chance event, based mainly on influencing the access of the two types of sperm to the egg so as to give one or the other the greater chance of successful entry. None of these schemes has so far been notably effective, although some quantitative effects have been reported (6). External human fertilization provides another opportunity, primarily because of the window it opens on fertilized eggs in preimplantation stages. Suppose it were possible to distinguish XX and XY eggs or early embryos by some noninjurious technique. It is possible to distinguish XX and XY cells at later stages because one of the X chromosomes becomes inactive in the female and enlarges to form the visible Barr body. This "marker" can be detected in embryonic cells obtained by amniocentesis, presenting the somewhat unhappy opportunity of aborting the unwanted sex type. But if in some way detection could be accomplished prior to implantation (the visible difference appears at about implantation), the unwanted sex type could be discarded without initiating pregnancy. This is ethically unacceptable in some value systems but clearly seems preferable, by any value system, to a later-stage abortion.

There would, however, be other issues involved in utilizing this option even if it became technically feasible. A particular question often discussed is whether such sex selection, whatever the technique, might tilt the approximately equal balance of the natural sex ratio. This could have significant demographic and social consequences, and possibly unfortunate ones. Clearly, the relationshps between individual free choice and broader social purpose would need careful consideration in establishing policy. Sex selection, however, is only one example of the kind of options that may be presented by external fertilization. The dissimilarity of X and Y is an instance of a visible chromosomal difference that is significant developmentally. Reference has been made to the high rate of loss of human embryos prior to implantation. Many of the embryos lost are believed to be genetically defective and to have visible chromosomal defects. A few of the less defective ones successfully implant and turn up later with postnatal abnormalities accompanied by atypical chromosomal shape or function. These might be detected by preimplantation examination externally.

Although there is legitimate concern that external fertilization may *increase* the frequency of genetic abnormality, there is also the possibility that the process can *reduce* this frequency by providing more effective screening prior to implantation than does the natural process.

These two possibilities—screening for sex type and for genetic defects—represent possible interventions that do not alter the properties of the developing embryo. There are a number of interventions of possible advantage that *would* alter embryonic properties, either for test purposes or to influence the resulting offspring. In testing, the presumed intention would not be to implant the embryo but to discard it before it could become sentient. The intention might be, for example, to get more precise information about suspected toxicities. A number of chemical agents have come under suspicion as deleterious to developing human embryos, particularly in stages of organ formation. Tests on animals and other living systems may give a strong indication of such embryonic toxicity, but, particularly where effects are weak and yet significant, uncertainty persists in the absence of direct demonstration on human embryos themselves. This, unfortunately, is sometimes provided inadvertently—as in the thalidomide tragedy. It would be useful to have nonsentient human test systems for avoiding damaged lives. Whether this usefulness would outweigh other considerations is a matter for the most searching examination in light of overall purposes.

Intervention To Affect Offspring

Intervention deliberately to alter embryonic properties in ways that *will* have consequence in offspring certainly is the most controversial of possibilities and, indeed, has colored the whole discussion of external human fertilization. In raising the matter it should be clear that it probably is not an early prospect, that it is not a *necessary* sequel (and may not even be a possible one), and that to discuss it is not necessarily to advocate it.

Several kinds of intervention should be distinguished: (1) repair of genetic defect; (2) genetic modification; (3) developmental or epigenetic modification. Repair of genetic defect was referred to in Chapter III. Genetic defect designates abnormality or disease initiated by a specific genetic alteration. A large number of such defects are now known, and some have been traced from a particular altered gene (a segment of DNA of specific sequence) through a particular altered protein (of specific amino acid sequence) to a particular symptom. The classic case is human sickle cell anemia. Repair of this genetic defect, rather than therapy for its effect, means that the abnormal DNA sequence is altered or replaced so as to restore the capability to make the normal protein. If this is done in somatic cells, the repair is effective in the individual treated but is not passed on to offspring. If it is done so as to alter germinal cells (sperm- or egg-producing), the effect is truly genetic—that is, it is transmissible indefinitely through generations.

It is the possibility of the last effect that is specifically opened by external fertilization. The inner cell mass of the blastocyst is the precursor to all cells of the embryo proper. If the genetic constitution of a significant number of its cells were suitably changed, so, too, might be that of the germinal cells that give rise to sperm and eggs. Such an effect has been reported in chimeras produced by embryo fusion (Chapter III). Genetic change in cells themselves might be accomplished in several ways, no one of which has yet been shown to work. The best candidate would seem to be the addition of isolated normal human genes for a required protein—for example, globin genes. These genes have now been identified and can be made in considerable quantity by replication in bacteria by means of recombinant DNA techniques. Direct exposure of inner cell masses to this DNA, as judged from other results, should lead to some uptake and incorporation into the DNA of the target cells. Efficiency of the process is low, however, meaning that only a small percentage of the cells might be affected. Greater efficiency would be expected if the globin genes were recombined with DNA of a suitable virus that penetrates cell membranes and deposits its DNA into that of host cells. Obviously there is still much research required with mouse embryos before this new technique could be applied to humans. Nonetheless, motivation would be strong if, for example, the procedure could reduce the number of individuals, primarily blacks, carrying or manifesting the defective gene for sickle cell anemia.

Genetic modification, rather than repair of genetic defect, takes us a step further in possible impact and controversy. Repairing a defect that leads to a life-crippling disease is clearly a desirable objective. Modifying normal genes or adding new ones to "improve" individuals or the species is quite another matter. Fortunately, it is also considerably more difficult in both theory and practice and, hence, considerably further down the road in terms of priority even of serious consideration. There is, however, an essential point to be made. The classic case of sickle cell anemia, profoundly instructive and important though it is, belongs to a special category of unusually direct relationship between genetic determinant and fully developed property. In most instances, particularly when such characteristics of great human interest as beauty, personality, and intelligence are involved, the relationship is far more complex than that between one gene and one protein. Most such characteristics are affected by many genes. Moreover, most genes have effects on more than one characteristic. The notion, therefore, that genetic intervention is likely to be used for planned changes in general aspects of human nature—whether for better or for worse—is a gross overassessment of any realistic current potential. As we approach 1984, whatever it may bring, we are acquiring an enhanced capability to deal with genetic disease, but we can be certain that human beings will not yet be constructed from our own genetic blueprints—not in 1984 nor in any reasonably foreseeable future.

Developmental Intervention—Cloning

In fact, we may be closer to a capability for more substantial intervention of the third kind—developmental or epigenetic. To be sure, interventions of the second and third kind overlap in some degree. Replacement of the nucleus of a frog fusion-cell with one from a later-stage individual is a developmental manipulation, but it has genetic consequences. If the fusion-cell continues development, it will show the genetic characteristics of the implanted nucleus. The purpose of the transfer, however, is to find out whether later-stage nuclei are so altered by developmental progression that they can no longer function like the fusion-nucleus from which they were derived. The question has theoretical interest, but it also offers a possible basis for what has been much discussed in recent years—human cloning. If the nucleus-donor were an adult and the nucleus functioned normally, the offspring would be genetically identical with the donor—a clone. The relation between the donor and recipient would be that of identical twins—except that they would be of successive generations. We have no kinship designation for such a relationship—in one sense they would be siblings, in another sense parent and child. The bizarreness of the relationship is what apparently generates interest.

What is the technical possibility of producing such a human clone? The actual physical manipulation has been carried out in frogs and, recently, in the mouse. In the best analyzed case, the frog (or toad), there is no question but that nuclei from embryonic stages can be returned to the fusion-cell, where they will function to produce a normal embryo. There is considerable question whether nuclei from adults can do the same thing and, if they cannot, why they cannot. It may be that nuclei from some kinds of adult cells can, but some cannot. It may also be that some nuclei that cannot function as fusion-nuclei when transferred directly to a fusion-cell could be conditioned to do so by first transferring them to developing eggs. It may also be that nuclei from such adult cells as spermatogonia—cells that will become sperm but have not yet reduced their chromosomal complement from diploid to haploid—would be specially capable of functioning in place of the fusion-cell nucleus. These are all questions to be further investigated in frogs and mice, for their theoretical interest and their possible practical usefulness in animal husbandry.

Their value in animal husbandry lies in the possibility that means may be found to preserve a particularly favorable genetic constitution—by asexual reproduction. The sexual process always leads to new and varied genetic constitutions; that is its great strength evolutionarily. But, even in nature, asexual processes also have an advantage; many plants propagate asexually (as clones), most of the time by forming runners that produce new individuals of identical genetic constitution. Higher animals do not have this capacity, but nuclear transplantation can provide the equivalent, if there is an advantage to be gained. A prize breed of cattle that produces an especially desirable individual is a likely selection for such an advantage. Another example is an unusually successful race horse. To breed such individuals sexually in order to continue a line is a gamble. The offspring will vary, combining in varying ways the traits of the unusual parent and the mate. This is genetic roulette, the inevitable consequence of the sexual process. If you have an individual whose *complete* genetic identity you wish to preserve, the effective process of choice is cloning by nuclear transfer.

If cloning were worked out in mice and shown to be successful in cattle and horses, would it work in humans? The best guess, scientifically, is that it probably would work, if the logistical problem of getting enough eggs and suitable donor nuclei could be solved. The technological question, therefore, probably is to be answered affirmatively; it could be made to work, if it were an important objective. Whether it *should* be made to work is an entirely different question, one that needs at least equally careful thought. The key issue appears to be the *purpose* involved and the likelihood of achieving that purpose without unwanted side effects.

In cattle and horses, the purpose in both cases is to preserve a particularly desirable genetic constitution. In cattle, a particularly desirable characteristic is high muscle-to-bone ratio, since it is primarily in muscle that economic and nutritional value reside. Other desirable characteristics are disease resistance, ability to use energy-conserving fodders, water requirement, etc. Such characteristics are likely to be transferred biologically, so the purpose has a good chance of being achieved. There is, however, a caveat. Cloning is not a one-time procedure; it must be repeated in each generation if the genetic constitution is to be preserved. The logistics and economics of scaling up the process to yield thousands of identical cattle need careful analysis. Moreover, the result would be genetically homogeneous herds, presumably all female. What then happens if circumstances change? If new cattle disease to which this genetic constitution is especially susceptible erupts, would genetic homogeneity then entirely defeat the initial purpose?

The race horse case is a little different, and in interesting ways. The purpose is apparently the same, to propagate a particular genetic constitution. But the especially desirable characteristic is winning races. Is this determined entirely biologically by genetic constitution? Or do trainers and jockeys play at least a contributory role? If they do not, what would the race be like if all ten entries were of the same genetic constitution? Would there, in fact, be a race that would stir interest and excitement? Would cloning of race horses on any large scale not be self-defeating? If the process were limited to generating only one clonal descendant of each successful race horse, would we see the same races run over and over again? Does genetic roulette not, in fact, better serve the recreational and even economic aspects of horse-racing?

The human case is, of course, still more complex when it comes to defining the purpose to be served and the probability of realizing it. Despite great interest in the concept of human cloning, there has been no thoughtful discussion of the purposes to be sought, the probability of achieving them, or the unanticipated by-products that may be involved. Once again, the general purpose is to reproduce a particular genetic constitution. Suggested scenarios justifying the general purpose, however, are very different in implications.

One may be called the egotistical scenario, the desire of an individual to create another "in his own image" without the contaminating contribution of a biological mate. That there are individuals who might be so motivated is not inconceivable. Should a limited number of individuals accomplish their objective and achieve their own psychological satisfaction, it is hard to see what harm would be done, other than to the individuals involved. The best guess scientifically would be that the product of cloning would be less like the source than would be two identical twins. Strictly biological characteristics would be quite similar or identical. For example, blood, skin, kidney, or heart transplantation between the two should not encounter immunological resistance. General physical features should show considerable resemblance at comparable stages, but, with advancing age, greater divergence might be expected than in identical twins, since exposures would be to different time-frames. In the particularly significant matter of personal identity and psychological and social characteristics, however, the divergence due to differing time-frames would be expected to produce much greater differences than in identical twins. There is good reason to doubt that the donor would necessarily recognize or take satisfaction from "his own image." This is, of course, because the relation between genetic constitution and psychological and social identity is so extremely complex and, accordingly, so labile.

A second scenario may be called the social benefit scenario, and it, too, may be examined on either the cattle or the horse model. On the cattle model it suggests that, if a successful, respected, or admired person—in any of the dimensions by which this may be measured—occurs in the population, there is a social benefit in making multiple genetic copies of that person. Implicit are the assumptions that genetic copies have a high probability of also being successful, respected, or admired (multiple Einsteins is the usual example); that if one is good, many are cumulatively better (a homogeneous generation of Einsteins); and that the human species of the future can be mightily improved in this way (Einsteins forever). Application of the cattle model to humans requires at least similar reservations to those expressed for cattle, and even deeper reservations are easily imagined.

The horse model corrects some of the crudities of the cattle model. It recognizes that for the human race greater variety of types is desirable (add to multiple Einsteins, other multiple desirables); that if some percentage of successful, respected, or admired people in a generation is good, it would be still better if everyone were successful, respected, or admired (a homogenous generation of success, respect, and admiration); and that the human species could be elevated in this way (winners all and forever). The reservations expressed about the horse model for horses pertain also for humans, and, again, even deeper reservations are easily imagined.

The third scenario may be called the social disbenefit scenario. It recognizes the same potential in replication of particular human genetic constitutions but applies that potential in the interest of a powerful individual or collective elite—whether the corporate establishment or a malign dictatorship. Here the clones are either selected from variants in the existing population that have suitable characteristics—docility, strength, capacity to endure monotony, programmability, etc.—or these are created by other genetic manipulations and stabilized by cloning. In either event, cloning becomes the means for perpetuating a society based on fixed caste, with only the upper stratum leading privileged lives of excitement, freedom, and luxury. The possibility that such abuse of cloning might occur is considered an argument against its use for any purpose and even against its use in research. The argument is that the existence of cloning will strengthen tendencies toward autocratic forms of society, and a slide toward the anthill. In fact, it seems that autocratic societies would have to exist first in order to initiate cloning as a repressive social ordering device.

Other Developmental Interventions

The process known as artificial parthenogenesis might be combined with cloning to yield further consequences. Cloning is possible with female as well as with male diploid nuclei, including a diploid nucleus from the egg donor. In the last case the product would be a female twin of the egg donor. By continued and exclusive application of the technique, an almost totally female and genetically homogeneous society could be created and perpetuated. The number of required males, as in the case of breeding bulls, would only have to be sufficient to provide sperm to activate the eggs. Even that requirement could be eliminated if human eggs could be activated parthenogenetically. This occurs naturally in many animals but not regularly in any mammals. It can also be induced artificially in frogs and some mammals but with no normal offspring so far resulting in the latter case. If it could be accomplished externally, regularly, and reliably on human eggs, it would open at least a formal option for a totally female society.

The process of diploidization, recently reported in mice, affords another route in the same direction but with even more drastic genetic consequences. The procedure does not clone an existing genetic constitution but creates a cloneable new one of a rather special kind. Diploidization is accomplished in the following way. Following sperm entry, resulting in activation of the development of the egg, there briefly are two "pronuclei" in the egg—its own and that of the sperm. If one of these is removed and the egg is treated with an appropriate chemical, its first division can be inhibited until the remaining nucleus has undergone chromosomal duplication. If the inhibiting chemical is then washed away, the egg will begin a new division cycle. The nucleus, now having a duplicated or diploid set of chromosomes, reduplicates them again and undergoes typical mitosis, giving to each daughter cell a complete double set of chromosomes.

The consequence of this intervention is that the egg nucleus, if diploidization were carried out on a human egg, would have 23 pairs of *identical* chromosomes, since each pair was derived by duplication of a maternal or paternal chromosome. If the egg went on to normal development, it would have to be female, since a YY fusion-cell would be produced if the sperm pronucleus remained in the egg and YY is inviable. However, a number of other eggs would also be inviable, because the procedure would have made the fusion-cell totally homozygous; that is, every gene would have an identical counterpart instead of a possibly different one from the opposite parent. In this case every recessive gene would be expressed, including the three to five recessive lethals known to be present statistically in each individual human being. This means that the eggs that survive this procedure would be free of recessive lethals but might be weakened by additional sublethal recessives. A truly vigorous individual produced in this way would be unusual indeed, having been genetically "sanitized" of most deleterious recessives and able to be cloned in that state. Such "sanitized" females mating with normal males would have offspring whose variability would only be half that of usual matings and the residual variety would entirely reflect heterozygosity of the male. Repetition of the process through several cycles of cloning on both sides could produce highly "inbred" individuals with relatively constant characteristics maintained even in sexual reproduction. Graft rejection, for example, might be eliminated by such a process—along with much else of the genetically derived variety we associate with current humanness.

What this state would be like if, in fact, it were to be achieved is truly impossible to forecast. The only point in raising it as a possibility at the present time is to emphasize two things: (1) we are currently acquiring biological capabilities that at least open options in these directions; and (2) we should at least give consideration to whether we wish to *drift* along these paths or whether we wish to introduce *deliberate purpose* as a factor.

The Policy Process

Is there anything special about the issues we have been discussing? If so, does it impose special requirements on the way we formulate policy? Are current mechanisms for policy formation and decision-making adequate to the task? What new mechanisms or modifications of old mechanisms may be necessary?

There *is* something special about the choices now before us. For example, they are of our own making. They are not—like earthquakes, hurricanes, or cancer—visited upon us. The choices have been self-created, through deliberate scientific effort. Nor were we taken totally unawares. The development of external human fertilization has been a specific objective of a small but dedicated group of investigators for over a decade. Its desirability, feasibility, and even ethics were discussed in both scientific and lay publications for a good part of the period of development. In a sense a policy decision to go ahead with it was reached, over strongly stated objections of a few critics, by the resolve of biomedical scientists and the tacit acceptance of the general community.

If we brought ourselves to this point, it would appear that we could lay the matter aside unused or make decisions as to exactly where we want to go. It turns out, however, not to be quite that simple. Mixed with foreseen problems are foreseen benefits. To some, the problems outweigh the benefits; to others, it is vice versa. To still others, problems and benefits are not the issue; the whole business is anathema, even as a subject for discussion. What *we* want, collectively, is a matter of controversy. Meanwhile, the research process goes on—driven by other motivations—and options multiply.

The circumstances often are compared, implicitly or explicitly, with another technology we have created since midcentury—

one based upon nuclear energy. From it have come two of the most difficult problems of our times, the searing blast of the Bomb, and the insidious threat of disseminated radioactivity from the Bomb or from nuclear reactors and their wastes. In this case, too, we "decided" to proceed with scientific and technological initiative and, after initial phases of wartime secrecy, much public debate. In theory, after several decades of experience we could reverse the decision. In fact, international confrontation has locked us into the "benefit" of mutual deterrence—with escalating, diversifying, and proliferating nuclear weapons. And fast-depleting resources of fossil fuel have locked us into another benefit, at least partial dependence upon a nuclear alternative. It clearly is not easy to put a technological genie back into the bottle. And, if we could, would we accept the loss of the truly great benefits afforded by the use of radioactive materials for biological investigation and cancer therapy?

The options raised by external human fertilization, especially in combination with other advances, are numerous. They include possibilities that range widely in degree of imminence and level of consequence. Each needs its own analysis as to benefits, risks, and consequences. Nonetheless, taken together they raise profoundly important issues that need to be confronted as a whole. Given current trends of research generating new options for human intervention, do we passively await each new potential application and decide about it on its individual merits? Or do we anticipate developments so as to have a general policy to guide us when each issue arises? Shall this policy be such as to influence, positively or negatively, the probable rise of particular applications? Shall we attempt to formulate, in general but concrete terms, the purposes that are legitimate and illegitimate—to guide researchers in their efforts? Does such "steering" of advancing knowledge threaten the vigor and freedom of research?

It can be argued that not to consider these questions at this time is to fall unthinkingly into the first alternative of passive waiting. It is, however, a defensible course. There is a case to be made that forecasting of so broad a front of futures is impossible, with any reasonable degree of wisdom or capability for achieving and implementing concerted decisions. Besides, focusing attention on what at the moment may be only speculative possibilities invites sensationalism, excessive fears or anticipations, and possible unwarranted repression of the whole development. It is better, it can be argued, to let matters take their course, not to look for trouble, to deal with eventualities as they arise.

Yes, but we are at the beginning of a historic transformation—says a contrasting view—one that can go well or badly as recent precedents indicate. Without facing up to the general nature of the transformation, by relying on case-by-case decisions, we allow the trend to be set by short-term, narrow reasoning. Mistakes will be made, and these will color the entire enterprise. Better to lay down the gauntlet on the large issue—however it may be viewed—and to attempt to establish broad and effective principles on which to proceed. The new capabilities can be a great boon if handled carefully. They should not be lost to excessive concern about a repressive backlash.

Underlying these contrasting strategies is a deeper issue: Can anything now done make any real difference? Many opponents and proponents of scientific and technological advance share one conviction—the thrust of advance has a quality of the inexorable. Opponents view this quality as the product of strong coupling of science, technology, and the establishment (it does not today seem to matter whether the establishment is capitalist, socialist, or opportunistically mixed). Proponents view inexorability as the essential thrust to knowledge and application, rooted in intellectual curiosity and the desire to improve the human lot. To both groups the notion that developing technology can be steered by deliberate and concerted human purpose seems fanciful and naive.

This has brought forth the Cassandras who cry havoc. They insist that technology, brought into being to extend the powers and improve the lives of humanity, has developed a life of its own. It now dictates rather than serves human purpose. What *can* be done *will* be done by technologists—following their own eleventh commandment. Technology is the polluted wellspring of financial, military, and political malevolence, with science as handmaiden. Technology advances *on* humanity, as a destroyer not a servant. This rhetoric, exaggerated though it be, stirs echoes of concern in a public witnessing the obvious effects of overreaching technological application, both for war and for peace. The uncertain light of this technological dilemma raises special doubts about a process that is moving toward so vital a center, with all its emotional charge—the way in which we reproduce ourselves.

Moreover, external human fertilization is only an element in a larger and enlarging biotechnology, already palpable in agriculture and medicine, growing on the horizon in energy and materials production, and now, seemingly, turning its attention to human husbandry. The living world, and now the human experience, are the *materials* to be transformed by this technology. That is its special aspect. No point in saying, although accurately, that this is not entirely new. It is, nonetheless, becoming much more dramatic. External human fertilization is an obvious symbol that we—frail, flappable, and fallible—are taking life into our own hands, including our own humanity.

This is the special aspect of issues centering on external human fertilization, in turn layered upon the fundamental technological dilemma, so sharply epitomized by nuclear weaponry and the energy-yielding reactor. It is this specialness that imposes heavy burdens upon the required decision process. If we are to be *transformed*, we want a say in this, if in nothing else. We want to know *who* will be doing the transforming, for what *purpose*, and with what probable *consequence*. These are not unusual expectations in our form of society—in theory. But in practice our public life and our system of policy-making have become so complex, so opaque, so seemingly devious, that no one is sure who is deciding, with what purpose, and with what concern for each of us. The decision process in this highly consequential, and deeply personal, area must somehow cut across the maze of ordinary decision-making. It must clearly unite purpose, implementation, and consequence.

An Emerging Pattern

That is a tall order, but there are signs of movement to meet it. New mechanisms for policy formation are emerging out of concern that the older ways are not adequate for the task. Several factors have contributed. First is the increasing sensitivity already referred to, as science and technology have crept closer to the workings of persons and their inner selves. Second were the outrages perpetrated in the name of Nazi medicine and science that aroused the conscience of the Western World after the Second World War. These shameful episodes attracted attention to the need for protection of individuals against the asserted demands of "higher causes." The resulting Nurenberg Code became a model that was extended to more legitimate areas of medicine and science whenever individual rights had to be weighed against requirements for effective experimentation. Informed consent became a watchword for experiments involving human subjects *and* for patients in routine medical practice. Not only investigators but physicians and professionals in general have accepted a limitation on their "freedom" to pursue otherwise perfectly legitimate objectives at the expense of individual rights, a limitation backed by legal liability in the event that identifiable harm is done. Particularly significant is the fact that, in the United States, appropriate use of human subjects is overseen not by police or judicial authority but by "institutional committees" established for the specific purpose.

This leads to a third factor in the trend toward new mechanisms of decision-making in areas of sensitive technology. Because of the frequently strong scientific and technical content of the issues to be resolved, professional expertise is included as an essential element in decision-making. Moreover, because the matters are complex, no single kind of expertise usually is adequate. Institutional committees assessing the use of human subjects in experimentation involve not only a number of medical specialties but nonmedical professionals as well. Lawyers, religious leaders, and persons distinguished in public affairs often play important roles. Also, a new breed of "ethicists" has sprung up whose professional focus is centered on the knotty issues that regularly arise in both medical research and practice. Sufficient expertise must be assembled to yield a rounded perspective in any arena dealing with decisions on human rights and purposes.

A fourth factor is loosely referred to as public participation. In a representative democracy it was traditionally assumed that the public interest is registered through elected officials. Two facts, however, stand out clearly in the political reality of the United States today. Many citizens feel that their needs and desires are not being adequately expressed in the attitudes and actions of their elected representatives. Secondly, the number and range of public decisions far exceed the capability of individual elected representatives to deal soundly with all of them. Accordingly, a rich abundance of auxiliary mechanisms has sprung up around our official representative decision-making bodies. These mechanisms are intended to give more direct influence to individuals and groups of citizens. Some clearly serve "special interests"—that is, particular points of view are pressed to return benefit to the source. Others serve the "public interest," their activities being intended to return benefit to all citizens. Since there is not always agreement as to what constitutes benefit, the distinction between special and public interest is not always sharp. What is clear is that there is a growing number of means for more direct public participation, either by lobbying on the formal representational process or by creating additional, less formal decision-points.

The institutional review committees dealing with the use of human subjects in research are an example of auxiliary decision-points. They have their counterparts in dealing with issues relating both to recombinant DNA and to external human fertilization. With respect to recombinant DNA, the original guidelines established by the National Institutes of Health (NIH) called for the formation of institutional biohazard committees of mixed expertise. These were assigned the responsibility to review applications for support of research involving recombinant DNA and to ensure, on behalf of the sponsoring institution, observance of the guidelines. A subsequent revision modified these institutional committees, giving them greater local autonomy and strengthening their public representation. Similarly, the recombinant DNA advisory committee to the Director of the NIH, appointed to establish the guidelines, was continued under them as the national focus for further consideration of issues. Public nonexpert representation on the committee was increased by the same revision that affected local institutional committees. Moreover, throughout the process of establishing and revising the guidelines, the NIH Director encouraged the expression of public reaction and input to the process.

Meanwhile, debate in several local arenas (for example, Cambridge, Massachusetts; Princeton, New Jersey; San Diego, California) was channeled into similar advisory groups, made up partly of experts and partly of interested citizens. The reports of these groups, generally similar in substance, became the basis for such official local action as was taken. In only a few instances was actual legislation passed by formally representative bodies. The Congress held hearings and debated the matter in committees for the better part of two years but took no action. In effect, public policy-making was carried out through auxiliary mechanisms brought into existence for the specific purpose.

In effect, the same can be said of external human fertilization—so far as the matter has gone. While the Department of Health, Education and Welfare (DHEW) was drafting proposed policy, Congress created the National Commission for the Protection of Human Subjects. This was, in considerable part, a reaction to controversy centering on fetal research evolving out of the relaxation of abortion restrictions. The Commission's study and recommendations on fetal research did not specifically address external human fertilization, which at that time appeared to be on a distant horizon. Therefore, DHEW did not issue regulations but did stipulate that no research leading toward external fertilization would be funded without previous review by the Ethical Advisory Board. That Board, whose membership, as already noted, was diverse and included individuals with both substantive expertise and more general perspectives, was short-lived. Its function, however, was clearly as an auxiliary to an official decision-making body yet to be completed.

The pattern of these developments appears to reflect the recognition that the sensitivity and profundity of issues raised by such matters as individual rights in experimentation and capability to intervene genetically and developmentally in human reproduction are too weighty and too consequential to be considered adequately and wisely by our general political mechanisms. Experience with abortion policy has contributed to this recognition. Not only has a definitive and stable policy not evolved on the issue itself, but the combined legislative and judicial struggle has heavily contaminated other public policy areas. It is true that policy on so controversial a matter must ultimately be the product of a political process. That clearly does not say, however, that the soundest decision necessarily comes from the standard political mechanisms. Special auxiliary mechanisms may yield a less traumatic and ultimately more effective decision process.

A Possible New Mechanism

What would be the desirable features of such a mechanism? Three features arise out of what already has been said: (1) credibility and dignity that match the sensitivity and profundity of the subject; (2) a suitable ensemble of essential expertise; (3) appropriate public access and participation. The need for credibility and dignity in the decision process cannot be too strongly emphasized. We should at least consider that we may be moving toward an epic transformation in human reproduction, bringing this central biological process under greater human control. Perhaps this is not true, and perhaps there is nothing to be done if it is. But perhaps, also, the transformation is coming, and perhaps it can be eased and influenced as to nature and timing so as to be more expressive of our highest sense of purpose and objective. Whatever the conclusion, we should reach it in a way that commands general respect and can be regarded with pride by future generations. Will this be the case if it happens almost by accident because of inadequate focus and narrow perspective?

Public access and participation also need further brief comment. A distinction does have to be made between *access* and *participation*. In the socially and politically complex society we have created, there is no conceivable mechanism by which every citizen can participate fully in every public decision. Even given the information and communications revolutions now in process, there can never be, nor would anyone want, a continuous town meeting of the United States as a primary mechanism of decision- or policy-making. In reality, each issue has what has been called its attentive public. For some issues it is large, and for some quite small. It is not clear that efforts to make a particular attentive public larger would necessarily be socially productive. The important thing is to provide mechanisms to facilitate effective participation of the attentive public for a particular issue.

Something further is important, however. Whether attentive or not, no one wants, subsequent to a decision that affects him or her, to find that he or she was excluded. The decision process must admit every attentive person and assure that no inattentive person is denied opportunity to become attentive and a participant. Affording that opportunity is access, and access must be potentially universal if the decision process is to have credibility and to command general support.

These three points would make a good beginning. We do not yet have for external human fertilization and its possible sequelae a decision process that embodies all three. Yet there are additional features that would be desirable. These include continuity, phasing, effective impact, and international scope. We shall discuss each of them in order.

The options created by external human fertilization are likely to be presented successively over considerable time. They also, however, interact both in the issues they raise and in their possible effects and consequences. Therefore, with respect to particular purposes, consideration of sets of options may be more effective than consideration of individual ones, particularly as they might be taken up simply in order of immediacy and practical feasibility. This suggests that the appropriate deliberative mechanism should be long-term rather than short-term in duration, so as to provide comprehensiveness and continuity. It also suggests that the mechanism should function only for a special confined group of linked options rather than for a number of only secondarily related matters requiring repeated shift in focus.

Long-term continuity of deliberation also is conducive to phased policy- and decision-making—a desirable attribute when one is dealing with a changing and evolving phenomenon. A short-term mechanism is likely either to attempt to formulate an overall policy that may be premature, or to deal only with immediacies, making no provision for later further consideration. What seems needed is something in between—formulation of policy in steps or phases as the evolving situation unfolds. For example, opponents of the whole concept of external human fertilization cite future possible abuses as a basis for their opposition to steps that would yield admitted short-term benefits. There is no reason to believe that a phased policy with continued deliberation might not allow benefits to be realized in the near future while curtailing the possibility of later abuses. Moreover, the total set of conceivable options is staggering to many at this time and may provide a totally undigestible bolus for sound policy-making. If one takes up the matter only at its least difficult and most accessible margin, however, the passage of time for the accumulation of experience may allow the gradual resolution of some of the deeper and more difficult issues.

Given continuity and accepting the desirability of phased policy-making, there remains the problem of implementation of formulated policy. Here there are difficult questions that this discussion cannot fully answer. Instead, an effort will be made to clarify the difficulty and to propose a possible mechanism for discussion.

The problem is to decide where to place in our governance structure a mechanism whose function is primarily one of study and deliberation, but whose output, to be effective, must flow through channels whose authority can assure effective implementation. If such a mechanism is placed too deeply within the formal structure of government, it may be subject to bureaucratic blinders; if placed too far outside, it may be unable to assure consideration of its recommendations or their effective implementation.

In view of the rather considerable success of the National Commission for the Protection of Human Subjects, I am inclined to favor that experience as a model. A Special Presidential Commission on Intervention in Human Heredity and Development would provide essential dignity and stature. The Commission might have some fifteen members, ten selected for their relevant expertise, five for their high public standing and sensitivity to public attitudes. The Commission should be established by the Congress for an initial ten-year period, with individual appointments of five years, once renewable. The charge to the Commission should be (1) to review and monitor scientific and technological advances that may lead to hereditary or developmental human interventions; and (2) to make such recommendations as are deemed appropriate for policy with respect to these possible interventions. To accomplish its charge, the Commission should be empowered to carry out studies by its own staff or by others, to hold open public hearings in various parts of the country, and to publish reports. Its reports and recommendations, to be forthcoming not less often than once in each calendar year, should be made to the President and to the members of Congress. Where recommendations are made for action by executive agencies, heads of such agencies should be required to comment on these recommendations in the Federal Register within 90 days of their receipt, indicating and explaining their intended action. Recommendations for legislation would, of course, be referred to chairpersons of congressional committees and subcommittees with a request for comment.

A commission of this kind would meet the specifications listed for an effective deliberative mechanism. In its first five-year period it should be able to assess the general problem area, sort the issues, establish priorities, and initiate informed public discussion. Presumably, early tasks would be to complete the assessment and formation of policy with respect to clinical trials of external human fertilization and to consider the implications of application of the procedure to nonspousal situations. A longer-term task might involve consideration of the earliest time for assignment of partial or complete human rights to the developing embryo.

Establishment of a mechanism of this kind would have an additional impact. It would signal to the world community the interest and concern of the United States in the fundamental welfare of the human species. Just as the threat of nuclear holocaust, triggered conceivably by confrontation of only two nations, is worldwide, so possible deliberate modification of human heredity is of significance to all peoples. Although currently divided geographically, politically, ideologically, and ethnically, the worldwide human community has a single genetic pool. Watching patterns of human migration and of microbial epidemics, one can see signs of the enormously complicated ebb and flow in the oceans of genetic information shared around the world. Although the concept of One World has weakened in recent decades, the concept of One Species is unchallenged biologically and might renew our sense of human kinship. Any serious discussion of broader implications of external human fertilization should, therefore, be worldwide in scope. Our own first step in this direction should include a call for international participation.

Postscript

We have come to the end of a discussion of a preface—the advent of purposeful intervention in early human development. At a number of points in our discussion, purpose has come up as a critical factor in assessing the appropriateness of intervention. For example, to many people external fertilization is acceptable for the purpose of alleviating infertility of a married couple but not of an unmarried woman. Others might agree to both of these but would not accept as a legitimate purpose the production of early embryos to be experimented upon. Acceptability of purpose is an important determinant of acceptability of action. To some degree the end does justify the means in the real world—even if this should not be so in an ethically perfect one.

We cannot, therefore, leave this subject without some effort to clarify the matter of purpose as it relates to external human fertilization. I have used the term "acceptable social purpose" on several occasions. What does it mean, and how is it determined? I use the term to distinguish collective purpose from individual purpose. We know that individual purposes are sometimes not acceptable in justifying actions; we admonish children and punish criminals despite their pleas that their individual needs or desires led to their unacceptable acts. We call upon a higher social need as rationale for such impositions. For example, we say that individual actions may not disturb the peace or violate the rights of others. Social purpose, in this sense, is part political and part sociological. That individuals are called upon not to do what a consensus of their fellows object to is the political aspect. That individuals are constrained from disrupting the image and structure of the social collective is the sociological aspect. Taken together they constitute the thrust of "acceptable social purpose" as a standard for acceptable actions.

Acceptable social purpose is embodied in large part in tradition—whether of folklore, religion, law, or complex and indefinable social habit. Tradition is out of the past; it is codified experience, often dubiously equated with wisdom. Events and individuals in the present may be out of step with tradition. The friction between them then influences both. Traditions do change, grudgingly. Science, as a generator of new knowledge and change, is frequently involved in friction with tradition, especially when an advance of obvious social consequence occurs. We are witnessing such a case in external human fertilization. This, however, is an unusual case. It not only shakes up tradition derived from the past, but it calls for a "tradition" that is oriented toward the future. This is because among the issues raised by external fertilization is its possible impact upon the long-term human future—effects registered over generations and conceivably to achieve *intended* ends. To cope with this takes more than ordinary policy, it takes policy embodied in enduring tradition. We need not only a cumulative past-oriented tradition. We need to build upon that a *designed* future-operative tradition that encompasses broadly acceptable purposes.

Such a tradition, by definition, must provide consistent continuity. To command continuing adherence, it must be based upon the most widely shared human attributes, the essence of being human. To assure flexibility to meet a largely unknown future, it must emphasize principles not laws. To remain pertinent over generations it must not prejudge issues in contemporary terms but must rely heavily on cumulative future judgments. To be widely understood, it must be stated simply but cogently. These requirements will not be easily or quickly accomplished. But the process should begin, for what is sought requires an impact comparable in duration to that of the Ten Commandments or the Magna Carta.

What kinds of principles might be included in this future-operative tradition? First and foremost, a clear statement that the objective is to *preserve* and not to change humanity. Preserve must not be understood to mean opposition to all change, for absence of change is contrary to our history and clearly impossible in a universe in flux. If there were *no* human intervention, change would occur through the normal operation of genetic dynamics.

Preservation must be understood to mean the clarification, sharpening, and intensifying of human attributes, the opposite of diluting or transforming them. Cultivation, not designed transformation, is the objective.

A second principle, derivative from the first, might be that highest priority must be given to correction and elimination of the most obvious *defects*—those that clearly limit and curtail individual human potential. In present-day terms these two principles would justify the use of external fertilization to heighten the effectiveness of efforts to understand, alleviate, and eliminate the more frequent and disabling genetic and developmental abnormalities.

A third principle might be the converse of the second—that intervention would *never* be practiced with the intention of reducing or limiting individual human potential. This principle would exclude much-discussed and properly repugnant possible interventions intended to yield castes with biologically specialized and limited capabilities.

A fourth principle might be that interventions to satisfy individual needs or preferences without direct alteration of individual attributes (for example, sex selection) must be assessed in terms of collective purposes and possible consequences. This principle would require careful consideration and monitoring of the effects of interventions that allow human selection of any characteristics of offspring.

Clearly, other principles might be added. The intention here, however, is only to indicate that such clear specification of acceptable and unacceptable purposes, together with an effective means of ensuring that unacceptable purposes will not be pursued, would go far to relieve anxiety and to allow the more obviously constructive outcomes to be achieved.

Upon whom should responsibility rest for the formulation of such principles? Certainly it should have the early attention of the proposed Special Presidential Commission on Intervention in Human Heredity and Development, were it to come into existence. The Commission could provide important leadership and focus. However, it should be emphasized that professionals in a number of disciplines, as individuals and through their organizations and institutions, have an important role to play—both in the formulation of principles and in ensuring their implementation. Especially critical is the role of biomedical scientists and health practitioners. But almost equally important are social and behavioral scientists, ethicists, theologians, legal scholars, and other humanists. For it is hoped that this tradition for the future will not be primarily a matter of legislation, but rather one of widespread dedication of conscience. If that is to be so, if there is to be a new affirmation of the central importance of preserving, clarifying, and strengthening the attributes of humanness, the consequences may be even wider than defining the proper role of external human fertilization.

Addendum

So rapidly are matters moving that even while this book was in press significant new information became available about several matters discussed in these pages. A controversy erupted about the first clinical trials of genetic intervention in thallasemia (1), more details are reported in press accounts of nuclear transplants in mice (2), and both scientific papers and new press accounts have appeared dealing with continuing clinical trials of external human fertilization.

Edwards, Steptoe, and their colleagues at Oldham Hospital in Cambridge, England, have provided scientific reports (3) on the work that led to the two previously reported successful births. These resulted from 79 sterile women who were selected for treatment. Following timing of their menstrual cycles 45 of the 79 women yielded preovulatory eggs. 35 of these were fertilized successfully and 32 cleaved normally enough to be inserted into the uterus. Of the 32 women receiving cleaving embryos, four became pregnant but two aborted. Thus, the success rate was 6.3% of those receiving embryo transfers and 2.5% of those accepted for treatment. The Oldham-Cambridge group achieved few pregnancies and no live-births using gonadotropic stimulation prior to egg collection and subsequently relied entirely on natural menstrual cycles. Their most successful cases were with eggs obtained 24 hours after detection of an LH surge, cultured to the 8 or 16-cell stage and implanted into the uterus in the late evening.

A group in Melbourne, Australia, has been increasingly active in conducting clinical trials. Their first successful live-birth was reported in the press (4) as occurring on June 23, 1980, although the procedure and the occurrence of the pregnancy had been recorded in the scientific literature four months earlier (5). More recently, A. Lopata, a member of the group, summarized combined results of the Melbourne and Oldham-Cambridge groups, in a communication to *Nature* (6). He reported that their single successful live-birth was one of two pregnancies resulting from 14 embryo transfers carried out in 1979. Ten additional embryo transfers in the first half of 1980 yielded no additional pregnancies. Combining these data with those of the Oldham-Cambridge group, he calculates 11% efficiency in obtaining pregnancy after embryo transfer but only 3% in terms of resulting live births. This means that only 3 women in a hundred who have a developing embryo inserted into their uterus will bear a child. The fraction of those accepted for treatment is even lower and the fraction of those seeking treatment is lower still. Lopata outlines the many factors that may account for the low efficiency and comments that "systematic evaluation of all these factors is required before the next significant advance in human [external fertilization] and [embryo transfer] will be achieved."

An informal report appearing almost simultaneously (7) indicates that significant advance may already have been made. It briefly describes work by two other Melbourne investigators, Carl Wood and Alan Trounson, apparently working independently of the Lopata group. Whereas the Oldham-Cambridge and Lopata groups both reported lack of success when hormones were used to stimulate follicle development, Wood and Trounson found that as used by them it is very helpful. Not only did it simplify timing for obtaining preovulatory eggs but yielded multiple mature follicles. It was thus possible to implant two embryos in the uterus to increase the probability of success.

Wood and Trounson also modified the embryo insertion procedure in several ways that seem to have been favorable. Before these changes they had no successes in 60 insertions. After the changes 13 pregnancies were obtained in 103 women, and five of the pregnancies involved two embryos. Following some abortions, nine embryos at the time of the report were at the 8–24 week stage (generally a stable period) and four of the nine were twins. The overall efficiency for live-birth may be 7% for women having embryos inserted into their uterus—about twice that of earlier efforts.

These recent events signify several things relevant to policy discussion in the U.S. First, there are ample numbers of patients seeking help even at present low certainty of success. Second, investigation is continuing and significant improvements are being made. Third, the effort is likely to go forward elsewhere in the world regardless of national policy here. Our own decisions should take full cognizance of these facts.

REFERENCES

(1) See *New England Journal of Medicine* **303**: 1293–1300 (1980).

(2) Associated Press, Jan. 5, 1981; *The New York Times*, Jan. 8, 1981.

(3) Edwards, R. G., Steptoe, P. C. and Purdy, J. M., Establishing full-term human pregnancies using cleaving embryos grown *in vitro*. *Brit. J. Obst. Gynecol.* **87**: 737–756 (1980).

(4) United Press, June 24, 1980.

(5) Lopata, A., Johnston, I. W. H., Hoult, I. J. and Speirs, A. I., Pregnancy following intrauterine implantation of an embryo obtained by *in vitro* fertilization of a preovulatory egg. *Fert. Steril.* **33** 2: 117–120 (1980).

(6) Lopata, A., Successes and failures in human *in vitro* fertilization. *Nature* 288 (18/25 Dec.): 642–643 (1980).

(7) See *New Scientist*, 18/25 December 1980, p. 758.

Specific References

(1) In Ethics Advisory Board—HEW Support of Research Involving Human *in vitro* Fertilization and Embryo Transfer. Appendix, May 4, 1979, No. 8, p. 35 (1979). "EAB-Append." in subsequent citations refers to this same publication.

(2) Steptoe, P. C., and Edwards, R. G., Birth after reimplantation of a human embryo. *Lancet* **ii**, 366 (letter) (1978).

(3) Edwards, R. G., Fertilization of human eggs *in vitro*: Morals, ethics and the law. *Quart. Rev. Biol.* **49**:3–26 (1974).

(4) Mastroianni, L., in EAB, Append. No. 13, p. 7.

(5) Biggers, J. D., in EAB, Append. No. 8, pp. 7–18.

(6) Behrman, S. J., Artificial insemination and public policy. *New Eng. J. Med.* **500:** 619–620 (1979).

(7) Biggers, J. D., in EAB, Append. No. 8, p. 6.

(8) Hsu, Y-C., and Gonda, M. A., Monozygotic twin formation in mouse embryos *in vitro*. *Science* **209**: 605–606 (1980).

(9) Markert, C. L., and Petters, R. M., Manufactured hexaparental mice show that adults are derived from three embryonic cells. *Science* **202:** 56–58 (1978).

(10) Papaioannou, V., and Gardner, R. L., Investigation of the lethal yellow A^y/A^y embryo using mouse chimaeras. *J. Embryol. Exp. Morphol.* **52**: 153–163 (1979).

(11) Hsu, Y-C, *In vitro* development of individually cultured whole mouse embryos from blastocyst to early somite stage. *Develop. Biol.* **68**: 453–461 (1979).

(12) Cockroft, D. L., Nutrient requirements of rat embryos undergoing organogenesis *in vitro*. *J. Reprod. Fertil.* **57**: 505–510 (1979).

(13) Whittingham, D. G., Lyon, M. F., and Glenister, P. H., Long-term storage of mouse embryos at −196°C.: the effect of background radiation. *Genet. Res., Camb.* **29**: 171–181 (1977).

(14) Ilmensee, K., unpublished data, New York: reported in *Nature* **285**: 358 (1980).

(15) Rorvik, D. M., *In His Image*. New York: Lippincott (1978).

(16) Ilmensee, K., unpublished data, reported in *Science News,* **116**(4): **68** (1979), *Nature* **285**: 358 (1980).

(17) Shettles, L. B., Diploid nuclear replacement in mature human ova with cleavage. *Amer. J. Obstet. Gynecol.* **133**: 222–225 (1979).

(18) Cline, M. J., H. Stang, K. Mercola, L. Morse, R. Ruprecht, J. Browne, and W. Salser, Gene transfer in intact animals. *Nature* **284**: 422–425 (1980).

(19) Walters, L., Ethical issues in human *in vitro* fertilization and research involving early human embryos. In EAB, Suppl. No.. 1 Also *Hastings Center Report,* 23–24 (August, 1979).

(20) Kass, L. R., in EAB, Append. No. 2, p. 1.

(21) Kass, L. R., Making babies—the new biology and the "old" morality. *Public Interest* No. 26: 32–33 (1972).

(22) Fletcher, J., *The Ethics of Genetic Control: Ending Reproductive Roulette,* Garden City, New York: Anchor Books (1974).

(23) Ramsey, P., in EAB, Append. No. 7, pp. 14–15.

(24) Ramsey, P., in EAB, Append. No. 7, p. 21.

(25) Kass, L. R., in EAB, Append. No. 2, p. 16.

(26) Kass, L. R., in EAB, Append. No. 2, pp. 18–20.

(27) Ramsey, P., in EAB, Append. No. 7, p. 2.

(28) Gorowitz, S., in EAB, Append. No. 3, pp. 11–15.

(29) Roe vs. Wade, 410 US 113 (1973).

(30) Gorowitz, S., in EAB, Append. No. 3, p. 6.

(31) Gallup, G. G., Self-awareness in primates. *Amer. Sci.* 67 (4): 417–421 (1979).

(32) Popper, K. R., and Eccles, J. C., *The Self and Its Brain.* Berlin, New York: Springer (1977); Edelman, G. M., and Mountcastle, V. B., *The Mindful Brain.* Cambridge: MIT Press (1978).

(33) Biggers, J. D., in EAB, Append. No. 8, p. 10.

(34) Humphrey, T., Function of the nervous system during pre-natal life. In U. Stave (ed.), *Prenatal Physiology,* pp. 651–683. New York: Plenum (1978).

(35) Reinold, E., Ultrasonics in early pregnancy. Diagnostic scanning and fetal motor activity. *Contrib. Gynecol. Obstet.,* Vol. 1, p. 148 (1976).

(36) Carmichael, L., in P. H. Mussen (ed.), Carmichael's *Manual of Child Psychology,* pp. 447–563. New York: Wiley (1970).

(37) Globus, G. G., Maxwell, G., and Savodnik, I., *Consciousness and the Brain. A Scientific and Philosophical Inquiry.* New York: Plenum (1976).

(38) Purpura, D. P., Morphogenesis of visual cortex in the preterm infant. In Brazier, M. A. B. (ed.), *Growth and Development of the Brain.* New York: Raven Press, pp. 33–49 (1975).

(39) Gesell, A., *The Embryology of Behavior.* Westport, Connecticut: Greenwood Press (1971).

(40) Munn, N. L., The Evolution and Growth of Human Behavior. Boston: Houghton Mifflin (1965).

(41) Tanner, J. M., *Fetus into Man.* Cambridge, Mass.: Harvard Univ. Press (1978).

(42) Klass, D. W., and Daly, D. D. (editors), *Current Practice of Clinical Electroencephalography.* New York: Raven (1979).

(43) Marsh, F. H., and Self, D. J., *In vitro* fertilization at the Norfolk Clinic. Hastings Center Report 10(3): 5–6 (1980).

Appendix I

THE SECRETARY OF HEALTH, EDUCATION, AND WELFARE
WASHINGTON, D.C. 20201

September 15, 1978

MEMORANDUM FOR THE HONORABLE JAMES C. GAITHER
Chairman, The Ethics Advisory Board of HEW

In May, I referred to the Ethics Advisory Board an application that sought funds from the National Institutes of Health to perform research involving human *in vitro* fertilization. At that time the practical application of the research seemed years away. We have now seen the work of Professor Edwards and Mr. Steptoe in England, and the birth of an apparently normal child following *in vitro* fertilization of the mother's egg in the laboratory and transplantation of the embryo into the mother's womb.

This achievement has aroused great interest throughout the world. Research on *in vitro* fertilization and on embryo transplantation holds enormous promise. At the same time, it raises questions that reach to our most profound moral and ethical beliefs.

From a medical perspective, advancing our knowledge of reproductive biology may contribute to reducing genetic diseases and infant mortality, and to improving health in ways that we can only speculate about at the present time. In addition, perfection of the techniques of *in vitro* fertilization and embryo transplantation holds out the possibility that certain couples who cannot otherwise have children may now be able to have children of their own.

On the other hand, these procedures raise serious moral and ethical questions. Does the perfection of these techniques create a potential for abuse so severe that the Federal government should not support or should strictly limit its support of the research? Can techniques of *in vitro* fertilization and transplantation of the embryo damage the resulting fetus and lead to abnormal children? Will this research lead to selective breeding, to attempts to control the genetic makeup of offspring or to the use of "surrogate parents," where, for example, rich women might pay poor women to carry their children?

Additionally, despite the promise that this research holds, the very research process itself raises a panoply of questions about the rights and responsibilities of those involved. Are any of the participants -- such as the research investigator, the clinical practitioner, the hospital or university, the government funding agency -- legally liable for defects of a child conceived in the course of such research?

These scientific, ethical and legal issues must be thoroughly aired. We need to bring the best thinking this nation has to offer to bear on these subjects, and we must debate these questions publicly and openly. I would like the Ethics Advisory Board to address all the issues associated with in vitro fertilization and to provide recommendations on broad principles to guide the Department in future decision making.

I know the Board will conduct a thorough examination of these very important and extraordinarily difficult issues. You should solicit the widest possible public comment on these questions, involve knowledgeable and concerned members of the research community, consult thoroughly with ethicists and social and political representatives concerned with these questions, and assure that your review of this subject is given as wide public dissemination as possible.

Only through the widest possible public involvement and debate can we hope to reach a conclusion which can win the confidence and support of the American people on issues involving such basic ethical concerns. In the course of your consultations, you should arrange for public hearings throughout the nation -- in every HEW region -- to stimulate a national debate on this subject, and to assure that all interested parties have an opportunity to make their views known.

I appreciate the Board's assistance on these complex and sensitive issues and look forward to receiving your advice.

Joseph A. Califano, Jr.

Appendix II

Ethics Advisory Board

Department of Health,
Education, and Welfare

Report and Conclusions:

HEW Support of Research Involving Human *In Vitro* Fertilization and Embryo Transfer

---

May 4, 1979

ETHICS ADVISORY BOARD

CHAIRMAN: James C. Gaither, J.D.

VICE CHAIRMAN: David A. Hamburg, M.D.

Sissela Bok, Ph.D.
Lecturer in Medical Ethics
Harvard University

Jack T. Conway
Senior Vice President
United Way of America
Washington, D.C.

Henry W. Foster, M.D.
Professor and Chairman
Department of Obstetrics
and Gynecology
Meharry Medical College

James C. Gaither, J.D.
Cooley, Godward, Castro
Huddleson and Tatum
San Francisco, California

David A. Hamburg, M.D.
President, Institute of Medicine
National Academy of Sciences
Washington, D.C.

Donald A. Henderson, M.D.
Dean, School of Hygiene
and Public Health
Johns Hopkins University

Maurice Lazarus
Chairman, Finance Committee
Federated Department Stores, Inc.
Boston, Massachusetts

Richard A. McCormick, S.T.D.
Professor of Christian Ethics
Kennedy Institute for the Study
of Reproduction and Bioethics
Georgetown University

Robert F. Murray, M.D.
Chief, Division of
Medical Genetics
College of Medicine
Howard University

Mitchell W. Spellman, M.D.
Dean for Medical Services
and Professor of Surgery
Harvard Medical School

Daniel C. Tosteson, M.D.
Dean, Medical School
Harvard University

Agnes N. Williams, LL.B.
Potomac, Maryland

Eugene M. Zweiback, M.D.
Surgeon in Private Practice
Omaha, Nebraska

ETHICS ADVISORY BOARD STAFF

PROFESSIONAL STAFF

Charles R. McCarthy, Ph.D.
Staff Director

Barbara Mishkin, M.A.
Deputy Staff Director

F. William Dommel, Jr., J.D.
Special Assistant to the
Staff Director

Roy Branson, Ph.D.
Ethics

SPECIAL CONSULTANTS

Philip Halpern, J.D.
Legal Consultant to the
Chairman

LeRoy Walters, Ph.D.
Director, Center for Bioethics
Kennedy Institute
Georgetown University

SUPPORT STAFF

Roberta Garfinkle
Committee Assistant

Erma L. Pender

Coral M. Sweeney

Eleanor S. Yago

STUDENT ASSISTANTS

Jose Pertierra, M.A.

Ray Moseley, M.A.

Preface

Current regulations of the Department of Health, Education, and Welfare (HEW) prohibit the support of research involving the fertilization of a woman's egg (ovum) outside her body (*in vitro* fertilization) until the Ethics Advisory Board has advised the Secretary as to its ethical acceptability. In 1977, the Department received an application for support of such research and, after it has been approved from a scientific point of view, forward it to the Board. At its meeting in May 1978, the Board agreed to review the research proposal.

Over the summer, the announcement of the birth of a baby following *in vitro* fertilization in England aroused great public interest; it appears that a number of couples are ready and eager to avail themselves of such procedures in order to overcome infertility. Therefore, in September, Secretary Califano asked the Board to broaden its consideration of the pending application to include the scientific, ethical, legal and social issues surrounding human *in vitro* fertilization and embryo transfer in general.

This report is the result of over a half a year of study during which the Board asked scholars and experts in the fields of reproductive science, ethics, theology, law and the social sciences, to prepare reports and discuss the issues with Board members in public meetings. In addition, the Board held a series of eleven public hearings throughout the country in which private individuals, professional societies and public interest groups had an opportunity to present their views. The Board also received over 2,000 pieces of correspondence including letters, postcards and formal testimony, all of which were copied and distributed to each of the members.

Chapter I of the report provides background information about the human reproductive process and research involving *in vitro* fertilization and embryo transfer. Chapter II explores the technical and ethical issues surrounding such research in humans and Chapter III addresses the technical and ethical issues surrounding the use of the procedures in clinical practice. Chapter IV presents a review of the legal issues, and Chapter V summarizes public attitudes as presented to the board and as determined by recent public opinion polls. The Board's conclusions are set forth in Chapter VI.

The Board hopes that its deliberations and conclusions will be useful to the Secretary and staff of the Department in making decisions regarding the support and conduct of research involving human *in vitro* fertilization and embryo transfer.

* * * * *

An appendix containing papers prepared for the Board by scholars in the fields of reproductive science, ethics, theology, law, statistics, and social policy will be available through the U.S. Government Printing Office. Ordering information may be obtained from the Ethics Advisory Board, Westwood Building, Room 125, 5333 Westbard Avenue, Bethesda, Maryland 20016, telephone (301) 496–7776.

Chapter I—Background

A. *The Normal Human Reproductive Process*

Through long years of painstaking study reproductive biologists have been able to acquire significant information concerning the human reproductive process. The gathering of data on this process has presented formidable obstacles, since fertilization and the earliest days of embryonic development occur within the woman's body where, for both technical and ethical reasons, they are not readily accessible for scientific study.

According to the best available evidence, for the average couple the performance of the human reproductive system is only partially "efficient." That is, not every meeting of sperm and ovum results in the production of a viable embryo. One study estimates that in 16% of the cases where human ova are exposed to sperm, fertilizaiton fails to occur. When fertilization does occur, the rate of embryonic loss during the first week is estimated to be 18% and in the second week an additional 32%. According to this study, only 37% of human zygotes survive to be delivered subsequently as live infants.[1] Statistical surveys of the length of time generally required to establish a pregnancy seem to lend support to these estimates.[2]

These relatively high rates of embryonic loss are due in part to external environmental factors which impede continued embryonic development and in part to chromosomal or genetic abnormalities in the embryo itself. The exact proportion of embryonic loss due to each of these factors in unknown. However, one study estimates that perhaps 50% of the embryonic loss subsequent to successful fertilization is due to chromosomal aberrations.[3] Thus, natural selection against most embryos with serious chromosomal abnormalities seems to occur during pregnancy, particularly during the first eights weeks following fertilization.

B. *Previous Research With and Application of in Vitro Fertilization and/or Embryo Transfer*

1. General.—In previous research with humans and other species three major techniques have been employed: (a) *in vitro* fertilization without subsequent transfer of the embryo to the uterus of a female: (b) *in vitro* fertilization followed by embryo transfer; and (c) embryo transfer following fertilization by mating or artifical insemination. Only the first and second techniques have been employed with human beings.

For *in vitro* fertilization (in either the first or second cases listed above) a method must be found for harvesting ova from the female and for brining the ova into contact with sperm from the male in the laboratory setting. In human beings ova are usually secured from the female by means of a surgical procedure called laparoscopy. A needle is passed through the woman's navel and brought into proximity to one or both of her ovaries. Through visual sighting follicles containing mature ova are located, and the ova are removed from the follicles by means of the needle. Human females normally produce only one mature ovum per menstrual cyle; however, if certain hormones ar administered early in a given menstrual cycle, multiple ova are produced which can then be harvested during a single laparoscopic procedure.

Following the successful harvesting of ova, the ova and sperm from a male are placed in a laboratory medium where ova and sperm complete maturation and fertilization occurs. The early embryo is then transferred to a different laboratory medium for subsequent growth. In the first case noted above the embryo is retained in culture in the laboratory setting. In the second case the embryo is transferred to the uterus of a female—either the female donor of the ova or another female whose hormonal cycle is at approximately the same stage as the cycle of the donor female. If the transfer is successful, implantation and subsequent development of the embryo occur in the uterus of the recipient female.

In the third case fertilization occurs *in vivo* in the animal, either through mating or through artificial insemination. The ova may be either those of the inseminated female or those of a donor. Following fertilization but prior to implantation, the resulting embryo or embryos are removed from the reproductive tract of the female and are transferred to the reproductive tract(s) of one or more recipient females. If the transfer is successful, implantation and subsequent embryonic development occur in the recipient female(s).

In summary, the following combinations of *in vitro* fertilization and/or embryo transfer are possible:

i. *In vitro* fertilization without embryo transfer

ii. *In vitro* fertilization and subsequent embryo transfer

a. Transfer to the uterus of the donor

b. Transfer to the uterus of one or more other females

iii. *In vivo* fertilization and subsequent embryo transfer

a. Fertilization by means of mating

b. Fertilization by means of artificial insemination

c. Ova of the mated or inseminated female

d. Donor ova introduced into the female prior to fertilization.

2. Research and Applications with Animal Species.—a. Nonprimate Laboratory Animals. Successful laboratory experiments with embryo transfer of early rabbit embryos predated by almost 70 years the first successful experiment with *in vitro* fertilization. In 1890 Walter Heape—working in Cambridge, England—succeeded in transferring two embryos from an Angora doe rabbit which had been mated with an Angora buck into the oviduct of a Belgian hare doe which had itself mated several hours before. Six offspring were born to the Belgian hare doe, of which two were clearly Angoras.[4] A similar technique was applied to cultured mouse blastocysts in 1958 by Anne McClaren and John D. Biggers. Some of the offspring grew to adulthood and reproduced naturally to yield a second generation.[5]

Between 1930 and 1959 many investigators sought to imitate the process of embryonic development in the laboratory setting by means of *in vitro* fertilization. However, the researchers failed to devise sufficiently stringent criteria to demonstrate that early embryonic development was indeed the result of fertilization of ova by sperm rather than the effect of laboratory manipulation of the unfertilized ovum. (Severe trauma to the ovum, *e.g.*, puncture or electric shock, can in some cases induce cell division without fertilization. In 1959, however, M. C. Chang of the Worcester Foundation in Massachusetts succeeded in documenting *in vitro* fertilization in the rabbit by taking sperm from male rabbits with specific traits not present in the female ovum donor. The presence of the male traits in the offspring (following embryo transfer and subsequent development) provided unequivocal proof that the sperm had indeed transmitted genetic information to the offspring.[6]

Since 1933 there have been 5 published studies of embryo transfer following *in vivo* fertilization in rabbits, 3 in rats, and 1 in mice.[7] From 1959 to the present, 13 papers (including Chang's initial paper) on *in vitro* fertilization followed by embryo transfer in rabbits have been published, 8 papers on the same procedure in mice, and 1 in rats. In 3 of those studies, 1 on rats and 2 on rabbits, abnormal offspring were reported; however, the causes of the abnormalities are unknown.[8]

Many studies in experimental embryology do not include embryo transfer as a component; rather, they involve various types of laboratory investigation of the early embryo—whether produced by *in vivo* or *in vitro* fertilization. These non-transfer studies examine such topics as mechanisms of normal and abnormal fertilization; the earliest stages of embryonic development; causes of abnormality in early embryos; and the effect of various environmental factors, *e.g.*, radiation, freezing, and various chemicals, on fertilization and early development.[9] Research techniques employed in the study of these topics include fertilization *in vitro*; *in vitro* culture of early embryos to and beyond the blastocyst stage; the fusion of embryonic cells with other cells; the infection of embryonic cells with viruses; the introduction of various changes (chemical or temperature changes, for example) into the embryonic environment; biochemical studies of embryonic cells; and microscopic analysis of embryonic cells.[10]

The technique of superovulation—that is, the administration of a hormone which induces the female to produce a larger than usual number of ova—has sometimes been employed in conjunction with *in vitro* fertilization. Superovulation has been studied rather extensively in rabbits. In one controlled comparison of normally ovulated and superovulated oocytes (total number=538) 60.1% of embryos obtained following superovulation and 54.6% of those obtained following normal ovulation developed into normal young.[11] In contrast, several other studies in rabbits, as well as in mice, have concluded that an increase in the incidence of chromosomal aberrations occurs following superovulation.[12]

The effects of freezing mammalian embryos have also been studied in considerable detail. The most studied species is the mouse. In one study mouse embryos stored at $-195°$ C for 369 days were cultured and transferred after having been frozen and thawed. The freezing process caused some cellular damage, as evidenced by the fact that a smaller percentage of frozen embryos survived than did unfrozen controls. However, previously frozen offspring were normal and grew and reproduced at the same rate as control animals. The second-generation progeny of the frozen embryos were also normal.[13]

b. Farm Animals. In research with farm animals—particularly, cows, horses, sheep, goats, and pigs—the primary emphasis has been on application rather than on the development of basic knowledge. For this reason, more work has been done on embryo transfer following *in vivo* fertilization than on *in vitro* fertilization itself. Research both with *in vitro* fertilization and with embryo transfer is dwarfed by the use of artificial insemination for commercial breeding purposes: with the aid of artificial insemination no fewer than 100,000,000 cattle have been produced in the United States alone.[14]

Relatively little laboratory research with *in vitro* fertilization or with *in vivo* fertilization using donated ova has been performed in farm animals. Five successful studies in cattle, three in sheep, and one in pigs have been reported.[15]

In contrast, embryo transfer following *in vivo* fertilization of the female's own ova has been widely employed, primarily in cattle, during the past five years. Indeed, thousands of progeny have been produced by this method. Techniques for recovering early embryos from the female following fertilization include both surgical and nonsurgical means. Offspring from embryo transfer appear to be normal, although no carefully controlled study of the outcome of pregnancy has been undertaken.[16]

Two additional techniques which can be employed in conjunction with *in vitro* fertilization and/or embryo transfer have been studied in farm animals. In two studies efforts were made to evaluate the overall quality of early cattle embryos by examining them for compactness, symmetry, and density. These subjective qualitative assessments were successful in predicting differential rates of subsequent pregnancy.[17] A second technique which has been employed experimentally with cattle embryos is the determination of sex through removing cells from the trophoblastic layer of the early embryo. However, many embryos are damaged in the process of sex determination.[18]

c. Non-Human Primates. Relatively little research on *in vitro* fertilization and/or embryo transfer has been performed with non-human primates. Three studies beginning with that of Gould and associates in 1973[19] and continuing with the work of Dukelow and Kuehl[20] have demonstrated fertilization *in vitro* with the squirrel monkey. *In vitro* fertilization studies with the Olive baboon and the rhesus monkey have not yet provided definitive proof that fertilization has in fact occurred. However, in 1976 D. C. Kraemer and associates reported the successful transfer of an embryo from an Olive baboon to a synchronized female following *in vivo* fertilization.[21] Similarly, in 1977 J. H. Marston and associates reported a successful embryo transfer from one oviduct to the other in a female rhesus monkey after *in vivo* fertilization.[22]

The meager data from primate research may reflect technical and funding limitatons on the one hand, or a lack of interest or incentive on the other. Gould has noted that primate research is expensive and that the competition for research funds is a limiting factor. He further observes that investigators may be confronting "as yet unidentified problems regarding the culture requirements for successful maintenance on nonhuman primate gametes *in vitro.*"[23] By contrast, Sackett and Smith have expressed confidence that there would be no problem in obtaining a sufficient number of primates to undertake research in this area; further, they report that reliable normative data regarding fertilization, pregnancy, and early development exist against which to measure deviations from the norm resulting from *in vitro* fertilization and embryo transfer.[24]

3. Research and Applications in Humans.—Most successful human research has been concentratred on achieving *in vitro* fertilization and on culturing early human embryos in the laboratory. Efforts at clinical application of *in vitro* fertilization and embryo transfer to overcome infertility were notably unsuccessful until the latter half of 1978 and early 1979 when the delivery of three apparently healthy infants following these procedures was announced.

The first well documented achievement of *in vitro* fertilization with human gametes was reported in 1970 by R. G. Edwards, P. C. Steptoe, and J. M. Purdy.[25] Since 1970 there have been seven additional scientific reports of successful *in vitro* fertilization—four by R. G. Edwards and his colleagues,[26] two by A. Lopata and associates in Australia,[27] and one by Soupart and Strong in the United States.[28] No details concerning the apparently successful *in vitro* fertilization in Calcutta, India, have been published.

Embryo transfer in humans has been attempted only following *in vitro* fertilization. A total of three reports of such efforts have appeared in the scientific literature, one by the Australian group (in 1973),[29] and two by Edwards and Steptoe (in 1976 and 1978).[30] The first attempt led to raised levels of human chorionic gonadotropin in the maternal blood, but implantation was not documented. The second resulted in an ectopic pregnancy in one of the woman's Fallopian tubes. As is well known, the third reported attempt culminated in the birth of a female infant. In oral presentations to scientific meetings, Edwards and Steptoe have reported the birth of a second healthy child, a male, as well as the occurrence of spontaneous abortions in two additional pregnancies initiated by means of *in vitro* fertilization and embryo transfer. The four pregnancies reported by Edwards and Steptoe followed 32 attempts at embryo transfer.[31] In addition, the birth of a female child in India following *in vitro* fertilization and embryo transfer has been reported in the press.[32]

The potential risks of several aspects of human *in vitro* fertilization and embryo transfer have received some discussion in the scientific literature. The technique of superovulation is frequently (though not necessarily) employed in efforts to recover multiple oocytes for *in vitro* fertilization. One report indicates that the technique of superovulation may be associated with higher rates of a chromosomal abnormality (trisomy) in humans.[33] Similarly, evidence from research with mice suggest that too-high a concentration of sperm around the ovum *in vitro* may result in its fertilization by multiple sperm and thus lead to another type of abnormality (triploidy) in the embryo.[34]

In vitro fertilization techniques may also bypass a natural screening process to which sperm are subjected in human reproduction *in vitro*. There is some evidence to indicate that the female reproductive tract selectively eliminates many abnormal sperm. In one study of the human Fallopian tube, for example, it was demonstrated that few morphologically abnormal sperm reach the site of fertilization.[35] Similar observations have been made in studies of mice.[36] the extent of this risk, as well as the two types of risks noted in the preceding paragraph, is unknown.

Two other theoretical sources of risk to human embryos have not been documented in research performed to date: The risk of inducing point mutation or teratogenic effects in the early embryo.[37] The mammalian embryo is highly resistent to environmental insults. Massive insults generally kill rather than merely damage the preimplantation embryo.

These five types of potential risks in humans are, at present, either theoretical or hypothesized on the basis of rather limited data. In addition, even if superovulation or *in vitro* fertilization were to produce a chromosomally or genetically abnormal embryo, there is only a low probability that such an embryo would develop to term. The natural process by which most abnormal early embryos are lost during the early weeks of pregnancy would presumably be operative following *in vitro* fertilization, as well.

C. *The First Phase of the Ethical Debate*

Within the American context, the public debate concerning ethical aspects of *in vitro* fertilization was initiated by biologist James Watson. In an extended statement presented in January 1971 to the Panel on Science and Technology of the House Committee on Science and Astronautics, Watson expressed concern that research advances in human *in vitro* fertilization and the cloning of frogs could in the future lead to attemps to clone human beings.[38] Watson's views were given wide circulation through being excerpted in the May 1971 issue of Atlantic magazine.[39]

An essay defending *in vitro* fertilization appeared in *Nature* in May 1971—the same month that Watson's comments were published in the *Atlantic*. The *Nature* essay, written by British biologist R. G. Edwards and American lawyer David Sharpe, indicated potential benefits of *in vitro* fertilization research and advocated interdisciplinary consultation as the best method for social monitoring of the research.[40]

In late 1971 and the first half of 1972, ethical critiques of *in vitro* fertilization were eloquently presented by biologist-philosopher Leon Kass and theologian Paul Ramsey. The essays of Ramsey and Kass, published in leading medical and public-policy journals, questioned the means being employed in *in vitro* fertilization research and voiced concern about the potential future applications of the research.[41, 42] In announcing that it would publish the Ramsey essay, the *Journal of the American Medical Association* editorially called for a moratorium on human *in vitro* fertilization research.[43]

From mid-1972 to early 1974 relatively little ethical analysis of *in vitro* fertilization was published. A Ciba Foundation symposium on "The Law and Ethics of AID and Embryo Transfer" was held in 1972.[44] In an invitational symposium published in the November 1973 issue of the *Journal of Reproductive Medicine*, several authors—including veterinarian Banjamin Brackett, ethicist

Joseph Fletcher, and physicians Luigi Mastroianni and Landrum Shettles—presented sharply divergent viewpoints.[45] In addition, the Committee on the Life Sciences and Social Policy of the National Research Council, whose executive secretary was Leon Kass, completed a detailed technology assessment of *in vitro* fertilization in 1973. Publication of the report was delayed until 1977.[46]

In 1974 the ethical discussion of *in vitro* fertilization seemed to revive. Biologist R. G. Edwards published an extensive survey of medical, ethical, and legal questions surrounding the technique. Edwards devoted particular attention to answering the ethical objections which had previously been raised by Kass and Ramsey.[47] During the same year Joseph Fletcher published *The Ethics of Genetic Control.* In this work Fletcher affirmed the value, indeed the superiority, of numerous genetic and reproductive technologies, including *in vitro* fertilization, as compared with the conventional method of human reproduction.[48]

Between the publication of the National Research Council's technology assessment in 1975 and the middle of 1978 little new ethical literature on *in vitro* fertilization appeared. The first phase in the ethical debate in *in vitro* fertilization thus concluded with a pause. Not until the birth of a child conceived with the aid of the technique did the pause end and the second phase of the ethical debate begin.

D. *The Evoluation of HEW Involvement*

HEW involvement in setting guidelines for research involving *in vitro* fertilization and/or embryo transfer has resulted in the publication of three documents: A "draft working document of proposed policy" (November 16, 1973);[49] a set of proposed regulations (August 23, 1974);[50] and final regulations (August 8, 1975).[51] It is perhaps worthy of note that the questions of fetal research, research with pregnant women, and research involving children received substantially greater attention in the three HEW documents than did the issue of *in vitro* fertilization. This differential allocation of attention accurately reflected the public-policy setting of 1973, when fetal research, in particular, was a matter of significant public controversy. The relative de-emphasis of *in vitro* fertilization in the HEW guidelines also reflected the view that successful embryo transfer in humans was not likely to be technically feasible in the near future.

The successive versions of HEW guidelines and rules published between 1973 and 1975 tended toward less detail in their stipulations and toward a greater emphasis on a review procedure for proposed research with human *in vitro* fertilization and/or embryo transfer. The 1973 draft policy stipulated that:

1. "Care must be taken not to bring human ova fertilized *in vitro* to viability * * *"
2. "All proposals for research involving human *in vitro* fertilization must be reviewed by the Ethical Review Board."
3. "No research involving the implantation of human ova fertilized in the laboratory into recipient women should be supported until the appropriate scientific review boards are satisfied that there has been sufficient work in animals (including sub-human primates) to demonstrate the safety of the technique. It is recommended that this determination of safety include studies of natural born offspring of the products of *in vitro* fertilization."
4. "No implementation of human ova fertilized in the laboratory should be attempted until guidelines are developed governing the responsibilities of the donor and recipient 'parents' and of research institutions and personnel."[52]

In August 1974, subsequent to the passage of legislation establishing the National Commission for the Protection of Human Subjects but prior to the Commission's first meeting, HEW published proposed rule-making on research with several specific groups of human subjects. This document responded to comments on the November 16, 1973 preliminary draft regarding *in vitro* fertilization research, clarified the definition of a fetus, and suggested issues to be considered by the Ethical Advisory Board in its review of any proposed HEW supported research involving human *in vitro* fertilization or embryo transfer. In this 1974 document "fetus" was defined to include "both the product of *in vivo* conception and the product of *in vitro* fertilization which is subsequently implanted in the donor of the ovum."[53] With respect to unimplanted human embryos, the 1974 rules proposed no specific guidelines.

However, the 1974 HEW document recommended that the Ethical Advisory Board take into account certain issues in reviewing research proposals involving *in vitro* fertilization and/or embryo transfer:

With respect to the fertilization of human ova *in vitro*, it is expected that the Board will consider the extent to which current technology permits the continued development of such ova, as well as the legal and ethical issues surrounding the initiation and disposition of the products of such research.

With respect to implantation of fertilized human ova, it is expected that the Board will consider such factors as the safety of the technique (with respect to offspring) as demonstrated in animal studies, and clarification of the legal responsibilities of the donor and recipient parent(s) as well as the research personnel.[54]

In August 1975, Hew responded to the National Commission's report and recommendations concerning fetal research. Since the Commission had not specifically addressed the issue of research involving *in vitro* fertilization and/or embryo transfer, HEW chose not to promulgate substantive regulations governing such research. It did, however, clearly reiterate a procedural requirement:

(e) No application or proposal involving human *in vitro* fertilization may be funded by the Department or any component thereof until the application or proposal has been reviewed by the Ethical Advisory Board and the Board has rendered advice as to its acceptability from an ethical standpoint.[55]

The effect of this review requirement between August 1975 and September 1977, when the Ethics Advisory Board was appointed by HEW Secretary Califano, was to place a *de facto* moratorium on all HEW supported human research involving *in vitro* fertilization and/or embryo transfer.

Footnotes

1. Biggers, John D., *In Vitro* Fertilization, Embryo Culture and Embryo Transfer in the Human, a paper prepared for the Ethics Advisory Board, 1978, Table 2, p. 10, citing Leridon, H., Demographie des Echers de la Reproduction, in: Boue, A. and Thibault, C., eds., *Les Accidents Chromosomiques de la Reproduction*, Paris, Centre International de l'Enfance, 1973, pp. 13–27.

Biggers, *op. cit.*, p. 11, citing Roberts, C. J. and Lowe, C. R., Where Have all the Conceptions Gone?, *Lancet*, vol. i, pp. 498–499, 1975.

Biggers, *op. cit.*, p. 13, citing Boue, J. G. and Boue, A., Chromosomal Anomalies in Early Spontaneous Abortion, *Current Topics in Pathology*, vol. 62, 1976, pp. 193–208.

4. Biggers, *op. cit.*, p. 19, citing Heape, W., Preliminary Note on the Transplantation and Growth of Mammalian Ova with a Uterine Fostermother, *Proceedings of the Royal Society*, vol. 48, 1890, pp. 457–458.

5. Biggers, *op. cit.*, p. 19, citing McLaren, A. and Biggers, J. D., Successful Development and Birth of Mice Cultivated *In Vitro* as Early Embryos, *Nature*, vol. 182, 1959, pp. 877–878.

6. Biggers, *op. cit.*, p. 20, citing Chang, M. C., Fertilization of Rabbit Ova *In Vitro*, *Nature*, vol. 184, 1959, pp. 466–467.

7. Rice, Catherine, Supplement to: *In Vitro* Fertilization, Embryo Culture and Embryo Transfer in the Human by John D. Biggers, 1978, Table 1, pp. 1–6.

8. Biggers, *op. cit.*, Table 7, p. 40.

9. *Ibid.*, Table 3, p. 22; see also Walters, LeRoy, Ethical Issues in Human *In Vitro* Fertilization and Research Involving Early

Human Embryos, a paper prepared for the Ethics Advisory Board, 1978, p. 32, citing Fowler, Ruth E. and Edwards R. G., The Genetics of Early Human Development, in: Steinberg, Arthur G. and Bearn, Alexander G., eds., *Progress in Medical Genetics*, Vol. IX, New York, Grune and Stratton, 1973, pp. 92–95; Karp, L. E. and Donahue, R. P., preimplantational Ectogenesis—Science and Speculation Concerning In Vitro Fertilization and Related Procedures (Medical Progress), *Western Journal of Medicine*, vol. 124, p. 296, April 1976; National Research Council, Assembly of Behavioral and Social Sciences, Committee on the Life Sciences and Social Policy, *Assessing Biomedical Technologies: An Inquiry Into the Nature of the Process*, Washington, D.C., National Academy of Sciences, 1975, p. 27.

10. Culture of human embryos beyond the blastocyst stage has not yet been reported in the scientific literature. Walters, *op cit.*, p. 32. The use of several of these techniques in research with non-human embryos is described by Edwards, R. G., Fertilization of Human Eggs *In Vitro:* Morals, Ethics, and the Law, *Quarterly Review of Biology*, vol. 49, March, 1974, pp. 3–6.

11. Foote, Robert H., *In Vitro* Fertilization in Perspective, Relative to the Science and Art of Domestic Animal Reproduction, a paper prepared for the Ethics Advisory Board, 1978, p. 6, citing Maurer, R. R., Hunt, W. L., Van Vleck, L. D., and Foote, R. H., Developmental Potential of Superovulated Rabbit Ova, *Journal of Reproduction and Fertility*, vol. 15, 1968, pp. 171–175.

12. Biggers, *op cit.*, p. 33, citing Fujimoto, S., Pahlaven, N. and Dukelow, W. R., Chromosome Abnormalities in Rabbit Preimplantation Blastocysts Induced by Superovulation, *Journal of Reproduction and Fertility*, vol. 40, 1974, pp. 177–181; Fujimoto, S., Passantino, T. J., and Koenczoel, I., A Preliminary Note on Chromsome Abnormalities, in Intratubal Rabbit Embryos, *Proceedings of the Japanese Academy*, vol. 51, 1975, pp. 51–55; Takagi, N., and Sasaki, M., Digynic Triploidy After Superovulation in Mine, *Nature*, vol. 264, 1976, pp. 278–281; Maudlin, I., and Fraser, L.P., the Effect of PMSG Dose on the incidence of Chromosomal Anomalies in Mouse Embryos Fertilized *In Vitro*, *Journal of Reproduction and Fertility*, vol. 50, 1977, pp. 275–280.

Foote, *op cit.*, p. 16, citing Maurer, R.R., Bank, H., and Staples R.E., Pre- and Postnatal Development of Mouse Embryos After Storage for Different Periods at Cryogenic Temperatures, *Biology of Reproduction*, vol. 16, 1977, pp. 139–146.

14. Foote, *op cit.*, p. 5.

15. *Ibid.*, pp. 10–14.

16. *Ibid.*, p. 17, citing Betteridge, K.J., ed., *Embryo Transfer in Farm Animals*, Ottawa, Ontario, Canada Department of Agriculture, Monograph, vol. 16, 1977.

17. Foote, *op cit.*, p. 18, citing Shea, B.F., Hines, D. J., Lightfoot, D.E., Ollis, G.W., and Olson, S.M., The Transfer of Bovine Embryos, in: Rowson, L. E. A., ed., *Egg Transfer in Cattle*, Luxembourg, Commission of European Communities, EUR 5491, 1976, pp. 145–152; Elsden, R. P., Nelson, L. D., and Seidel, G. E., Jr., Superovulation of Cows with Follicle Stimulating Hormone and Pregnant Mare's Serum Gonadotropin, *Theriogenology*, vol. 9, 1978, pp. 17–26.

18. Foote, *op cit.*, p. 19, citing Hare, W. C. D. and Betteridge, K. H., Relationship of Embryo Sexing to Other Methods of Prenatal Sex Determination in Farm Animals: A Review, *Theriogenology*, vol. 9, 1978, pp. 27–43.

Gould, K. G., Fertilization *In Vitro* of Nonhuman Primate Ova: Present Status and Rationale for Further Development of the Technique, a paper prepared for the Ethics Advisory Board, 1978, p. 9, citing Gould, Cline, E. M. and Williams, W. L., Observation on the Introduction of Ovulation and Fertilization *In Vitro* in the Squirrel Monkey (Saimiri Sciureus), *Fertility and Sterility*, vol. 24, 1973, pp. 260–268.

20. Gould, *op cit.*, p. 9, citing Kuehl, T. J. and Dukelow, W. R., Ovulation Induction During the Anovulatory Season in Saimiri Sciureus, *Journal of Medical Primatology*, vol. 4, 1975, pp. 209–216; Dukelow, W. R. and Kuehl, T. J., in: Thibault, C., ed., *La Fecondation*, Paris, Masson, 1975, pp. 67–80.

21. Gould, *op cit.*, pp. 8–9, citing Kraemer, D.C., Moore, G. T., and Kramen, M. A., Babboon Infant Produced by Embryo Transfer, *Science*, vol. 192, 1976, pp. 1246–1247.

22. Gould, *op cit.*, pp. 7–8, citing Marston, J.H., Penn, R., and Sivelle, P.C., Successful Autotransfer of Tubal Eggs in the Rhesus Monkey (Macaca Mulatta), *Journal of Reproduction and Fertility*, vol. 49, 1977, pp. 175–176.

23. Gould, *op cit.*, p. 13.

24. Sackett, G.P., A Nonhuman Primate Research Model of Developmental Risk

Following *In Vitro* Fertilization and Embryo Transfer, a paper prepared for the Ethics Advisory Board, 1979.

25. Biggers, *op cit.*, p. 27, citing Edwards, R.G., Steptoe, P.C., and Purdy, J.M., Fertilization and Cleavage *In Vitro* of Preovular Human Oocytes, *Nature*, vol. 227, 1970, pp. 1307–1309.

26. Biggers, *op cit.*, pp. 27–28, citing Steptoe, P.C., Edwards, R.G., and Purdy, J.M., Human Blastocysts Grown in Culture, *Nature*, vol. 119, 1971, pp. 132–133; Steptoe, P.C., and Edwards, R.G., Preimplantation of a Human Embryo with Subsequent Tubal Pregnancy, *Lancet*, vol. i, 1976, pp. 880–882; Steptoe, P.C., and Edwards, R.G., Birth after the Reimplantation of a Human Embryo, *Lancet*, vol. ii, 1978, p. 336.

27. Biggers, *op cit.*, pp. 2, 29 citing DeKretzer, D., Dennis, P., Hudson, B., Leeton, J. Lopata, A., Outch, K., Talbot, J., and Wood, C., Transfer of a Human Zygote, *Lancet*, vol. ii, 1973, pp. 728–729; Lopata, A., McMaster, R., McBain, J.C., and Johnston, W.I.H., *In Vitro* Fertilization of Preovulatory Human Eggs, *Journal of Reproduction and Fertility*, vol. 52, 1978, pp. 339–342.

28. Biggers, *op. cit.*, pp. 30–31, citing Soupart, P. and Strong, P. A., Ultrastructural Observations on Human Oocytes Fertilized *In Vitro*, *Fertility and Sterility*, vol. 25, 1974, pp. 11–44.

29. Biggers, *op. cit.*, pp. 30–31, citing DeKretzer, *et al.*, Transfer of a Human Zygote, *Lancet*, vol. ii, 1973, pp. 728–729.

30. Biggers, *op. cit.*, p. 29, citing Steptoe, P. C., and Edwards, R. G., Reimplantation of a Human Embryo with Subsequent Tubal Pregnancy, *Lancet*, vol. i, 1976, pp. 880–882; Steptoe, P. C., and Edwards, R. G., Birth after the Reimplantation of a Human Embryo, *Lancet*, vol. ii, 1978, p. 366.

31. Short, R. V., Summary of the Presentation of Dr. P. C. Steptoe and Dr. R. G. Edwards at the Royal College of Obstetricians on Friday, January 26th, 1979, written report presented to the Ethics Advisory Board, February 2, 1979.

32. Test Tube Baby, World's Second, Born in India, *Washington Post*, October 6, 1978.

33. Biggers, *op. cit.*, p. 32, citing Boue, J. C., and Boue, A., Increased Frequency of Chromosomal Anomalies in Abortions After Induced Ovulation, *Lancet*, vol. i, 1973, p. 679.

34. Biggers, *op. cit.*, p. 33, citing Fraser, L. R., Zenellotti, H. M., Paton, G. R., and Drury, L. M., Increased Incidence of Triploidy in Embryos Derived from Mouse Eggs Fertilized *In Vitro*, *Nature*, vol. 260, 1976, pp. 39–40; Fraser, L. R., and Maudlin, L., Relationship Between Sperm Concentration and the Incidence of Polyspermy in Mouse Embryos Fertilized *In Vitro*, *Journal of Reproduction and Fertility*, vol. 52, 1978, pp. 103–106.

35. Biggers, *op. cit.*, p. 33, citing Ahlgren, M., Sperm Transport to and Survival in the Human Fallopian Tube, *Gynecologic Investigation*, vol. 6, 1975, pp. 200–214.

36. Biggers, *op. cit.*, citing Krzanowska, H., The Passage of Abnormal Spermatozoa Through the Uterotubal Junction of the Mouse, *Journal of Reproduction and Fertility*, vol. 38, 1974, pp. 81–90.

37. Biggers, *op. cit.*, pp. 33–35.

38. Watson, James D., Statement at the twelfth meeting of the Panel on Science and Technology, in *International Science Policy*, (Proceedings before the Committee on Science and Astronautics, U.S. House of Representatives, 92nd Congress, 1st Session, January 26, 27, and 28, 1971), Washington, D.C., U.S. Government Printing Office, 1971, pp. 336–344.

39. Watson, James D., Moving Toward Clonal Man: Is This What we Want? *Alantic*, vol. 227, 1971, pp. 50–53.

40. Edwards, Robert G., and Sharke, David J., Social Values and Research in Human Embryology, *Nature*, vol. 231, 1971, pp. 87–91.

41. Kass, Leon R., Babies by Means of *In Vitro* Fertilization: Unethical Experiments on the Unborn? *New England Journal of Medicine*, vol. 285, 1971, pp. 1174–1179; Kass Leon R., Making Babies—The New Biology and the "old" Morality, *Public Interest*, vol. 26, 1972, pp. 18–56.

42. Ramsey, Paul, Shall We 'Reproduce'?, *Journal of the American Medical Association*, vol. 220, 1972, pp. 1346–1350, 1480–1485.

43. Genetic Engineering in Man: Ethical Considerations (editorial), *Journal of the American Medical Association*, vol. 220, 1972, p. 721.

44. *Law and Ethics of A.I.D. and Embryo Transfer*, New York, American Elsevier, 1973.

45. Schumacher, Gebhard, F., *et al.*, *In Vitro* Fertilization of Human Ova and Blastocyst Transfer: An Invitational Symposium, *Journal of Reproductive Medicine*, vol. 11, 1973, pp. 192–200.

46. National Research Council, Assembly

of Behavioral and Social Sciences, Committee on the Life Sciences and Social Policy, *Assessing Biomedical Technologies: An Inquiry into the Nature of the Process,* Washington, D.C., National Academy of Sciences, 1975, pp. 13–31.

47. Edwards, R. G., Fertilization of Human Eggs *In Vitro*: Morals, Ethics and the Law, *Quarterly Review of Biology,* vol. 49, 1974, pp. 3–26.

48. Fletcher, Joseph, *The Ethics of Genetic Control: Ending Reproductive Roulette,* New York, Doubleday, 1974.

49. *Federal Register,* vol. 38, November 16, 1973, p. 31743.

50. *Federal Register,* vol. 39, August 23, 1974, p. 30650.

51. *Federal Register,* vol. 40, August 8, 1975, p. 33527.

52. *Federal Register,* vol. 38, November 16, 1973, p. 31743.

53. *Federal Register,* vol. 39, August 23, 1974, p. 30650

54. *Ibid.*

55. *Federal Register,* vol. 40, August 8, 1975, p. 33529.

Chapter II—Laboratory Research Involving Human In Vitro Fertilization and/or the Culture of Early Human Embryos: Technical and Ethical Issues

The technical and ethical issues surrounding *in vitro* Fertilization using human gametes depend, to some extent, on whether or not the procedure is performed with the intent of transferring the resulting embryos to women for further development. The discussion in this chapter relates to *in vitro* fertilization of human ova when there is no intention of transferring the product to establish a pregnancy. Chapter III deals with human *in vitro* fertilization performed with the specific intent of initiating a pregnancy.

These two chapters focus primary attention on technical and ethical issues as presented to the Ethics Advisory Board in papers prepared by its consultants. Thus, they do not summarize the primary scientific and ethical publications concerning *in vitro* fertilization and/or embryo transfer.

In one of the papers prepared at the request of the Board, LeRoy Walters surveyed the ethical literature on *in vitro* fertilization published through August 1978.[1] This survey noted that most of the ethical discussion on *in vitro* fertilization has concentrated on clinical applications of the technique (the topic of Chapter III) rather than on laboratory research with early human embryos (the topic of the present chapter). Central issues in the ethical literature on basic research with human embryos included the moral status of the early embryo, the need for such research, and the potential long-term consequences of the research. According to the same survey, commentators on ethical issues in the application of *in vitro* fertilization and/or embryo transfer discussed, among other topics, the need for *in vitro* fertilization as a method for overcoming infertility, the adequacy of prior laboratory and animal research, the risks of *in vitro* fertilization and embryo transfer to the ovum donor as well as to potential offspring, and the appropriateness of allocating scarce health care resources to the clinical application of such techniques. Many of these issues recurred in the papers presented to the Board, which are systematically reviewed in this and the following chapter.

A. The Goals and Potential Benefits of the Research. As noted in the preceding chapter many studies in experimental embryology do not include embryo transfer as a component. Several possible goals of laboratory research with human embryos have been identified:

1. Developing or testing more adequate contraceptives; [2]
2. Determining causes of infertility; [3]
3. Investigating the circumstances leading to the development of hyatidiform moles and their potential transformation into malignant tumors; [4]
4. Evaluating the effect of noxious agents or teratogens on the early embryo by means of an *in vitro* screening system; [5]
5. Studying the mechanisms by which

chromosomal abnormalities are produced; [6] and

6. Investigating the totipotential cells of very early embryos to increase understanding of normal and abnormal cell growth and differentiation.[7]

One additional potential goal of human *in vitro* fertilization and embryo culture is more controversial and therefore merits more detailed comment. R.V. Short suggests that a kind of *in vitro* assessment (or "toxicology testing") study might be performed to determine whether *in vitro* fertilization produces a higher incidence of embryonic abnormalities than the conventional *in vivo* method of human reproduction. In Short's view, if *in vitro* fertilization techniques do in fact lead to an excess of embryonic abnormalities, it would be preferable to discover that excess in the laboratory rather than at the time of amniocentesis or birth. Short argues that such a controlled *in vitro* study would also provide information concerning the probable success rate of *in vitro* fertilization.[8]

Several objections can be raised to such a proposal, as Short himself observes. First, there would be little basis for comparison following such a laboratory study since data concerning the incidence of abnormalities, particularly chromsomal abnormalities, in early human embryos following *in vivo* fertilization are quite limited. In fact, the totality of *in vivo* information relating to human preimplantation ova and embryos is "confined to 15 specimens, 9 recovered from the oviduct and 6 from the uterus." [9] At least two replies to this objection can be made. First, James Schlesselman notes that one can extrapolate statistically from three major studies of the incidence of chromosomal abnormalities following *in vivo* fertilization [10] that the natural incidence of such abnormalities in humans is between 396 per 1,000 and 477 per 1,000 at the time of implantation; prior to implantation the incidence of such abnormalities is presumably somewhat higher.[11] Schlesselman concludes that a 40–50% chromosomal abnormality rate in human embryos following *in vivo* fertilization is a reasonable baseline against which to compare the results of *in vitro* fertilization. A second reply is proposed by Short himself, who suggests that one could perform a controlled study of the actual incidence of embryonic defects following *in vivo* fertilization by flushing early embryos from the reproductive tracts of consenting volunteer research subjects. Short concedes that this aspect of the proposed risk-assessment study would present both medical and ethical difficulties of its own.[12]

A second possible objection to Short's proposal for a laboratory risk-assessment study is that it is unnecessary. This objection can take one of two forms. Schlesselman notes that for every 1,000 chromosomal abnormalities which are present in implanted blastocysts, only 5 to 7 survive to the point of live birth. Thus, 99.3% to 99.5% of chromosomally abnormal fetuses are eliminated *in vivo* through spontaneous abortion or fetal death. It follows, therefore, that even a doubling in the incidence of chromosomal abnormalities following *in vitro* fertilization—assuming that the technique or ancillary medical treatment did not facilitate the survival of abnormal embryos—would yield only an additional 6 to 7 chromosomally abnormal fetuses, which could, in Schlesselman's view, be detected by means of prenatal diagnosis and selectively aborted.[13]

An alternative argument against the necessity of Short's proposed risk-assessement study can be based on the essays of Biggers, who asserts that for the investigation of most questions concerning human reproduction a suitable animal model can be found. In his view, women should not be subjected to research risks and valuable human ova and embryos should not be used in research unless there is no reasonable alternative to a study in humans.[14]

Biggers' postion suggests a final issue to be considered under the rubric of goals and potential benefits of the research: How stringent a standard should be set with respect to the *need* for laboratory research on human *in vitro* fertilization and embryo transfer? There are three possible answers to this question. The least stringent standard would be that benefits can be expected from the human research. A somewhat more stringent standard would be that human research should hold out the prospect of more significant or more reliable benefits than research employing animal models.[15] The most stringent standard would require that the promised benefits of human research be achievable *only* through research using human gametes and early human embryos.

B. *The Design of the Research.* Biggers emphasizes that research on human *in vitro* fertilization and embryo culture, since it involves human volunteers, "should only be undertaken if efficiently designed experiments of adequate size are possible." [16] In his view, this stipulation may require that collaborative trials be conducted. Schlesselman's discussion of appropriate sample size for answering specific questions regarding human *in vitro* fertilization illustrates both the complexity of the design issue and the essential role of the biostatistician in helping to plan laboratory research with human gametes and embryos.[17]

C. *The Consent of Sperm and Ovum Donors.* Most discussion of the consent question for laboratory studies of *in vitro* fertilization has focused on the ovum donor. In most cases ova are harvested from women with intact ovaries by means of laparoscopy. The donation of ova may be associated with receiving hormones to induce superovulation and/or to mature the ova *in vivo* prior to harvest. In some cases ova are harvested at the same time that a tubal ligation is performed. There is unanimous agreement that the informed consent of ovum donors must be secured in advance of their participation as research subjects.[18] In addition, the particular vulnerability of infertility patients, who are dependent on the health professions for assistance in achieving pregnancy and who nonetheless may be asked to serve as ovum donors, has been noted in the literature on the consent question.[19]

Less thoroughly discussed are the issues of consent by semen donors and the use of ova excised from ovarian tissue removed for clinical reasons. Consent by semen donors might be particularly difficult to secure if semen were secured from a sperm bank rather than from a prospectively recruited donor. The view expressed in one published assessment of *in vitro* fertilization is that prior consent should be secured from all males whose sperm are to be used for *in vitro* fertilization.[20]

The harvesting of ova from excised ovarian tissue may prove to be inefficient from a purely practical standpoint unless hormone treatments are administered in advance of surgery. Prior consent to such hormone treatment would presumably be secured. However, even if ova were harvested from such tissue, without the previous administration of hormone to the female patient, gradually evolving general standards with respect to the use of human tissues for research purposes[21] would seem to suggest the necessity for securing the patient's consent to the use of her ova in laboratory research.

D. *The Status of the Early Human Embryo.* Two primary objections to laboratory research with human *in vitro* fertilization and embryo culture have been raised. The first is that such research is incompatible with the respect that is due to early human embryos. The second is that the potential adverse consequences of the research outweigh the potential benefits. These two objections will be discussed in the present and the succeeding section of this chapter.

The shape of the embryonic status question differs somewhat in the laboratory research context and the clinical context. As Leon Kass points out, many human embryos which would be studied in the laboratory would have been created solely for research purposes.[22] The major alternative would be to perform laboratory studies on untransferred embryos remaining after the fertilization of multiple ova and the transfer of only one to the uterus. However, from a research design standpoint total reliance on the use of untransferred embryos would seem to exclude research on the fertilization process and on the earliest stages of embryonic development.

At least three distinquishable answers to the embryonic-status question in the research context have been proposed. Kass himself, impressed by the continuities in embryonic and fetal development and by the potential viability of the early human embryo if it is transferred at the proper time, argues (1) that embryos ought not be deliberately created for research purposes[23] and (2) that no invasive or manipulative research should be performed on already-existing human embryos.[24] Any other policy would, according to Kass, symbolize the belief that early human embryos are "things or mere stuff." [25]

A second position on the embryonic-status is presented by Charles Curran, who argues that:

> From my ethical perspective truly human life is present two to three weeks after conception or shortly after the implantation of the embryo. Hence experimentation after that time and attempts to culture embryos *in vitro* beyond this stage raise insurmountable ethical problems.[26]

However, even for research involving the earliest stages of embryonic life Curran asserts that "[t]he nature of the matter involved in the research calls for respect and economy avoiding unnecessary waste." [27]
A similar position is articulated by Clifford Grobstein who suggests that "human cells, tissues and organs that have no reasonable prospect of possessing or developing sentient awareness" are "human materials rather than human beings or persons." Grobstein notes that "there are established practices for dealing with and disposing of human materials, practices that take into account the special status they have, having originated as human." [28] Grobstein's position is characterized as being similar rather than identical to Curran's for two reasons. First, it is not clear that Curran would extend his principle of respect to include non-embryonic human organs, tissues, or cells. Second, the criterion of possessing a potential for sentience seems not to be a part of Curran's position on embryonic status. Indeed, one could construe this criterion broadly to include all preimplantation embryos since, as Kass notes, they could be transferred, implanted, and develop to maturity; or one could interpret the criterion narrowly to exclude all preimplantation embryos since it is infeasible, given the current state of medical technology, to culture human embryos *in vitro* beyond the blastocyst stage.

A third position on embryonic status, represented by Samuel Gorovitz, adopts sentience (rather than the potential for sentience) as the primary criterion for determining the moral status of the human embryo or fetus in Gorovitz's view:

> The status of the embryo is not equivalent to that of a person, a child, an infant, or a fetus—at least a fetus from the point of development of the capacity for even primitive sentience.[29]

If by "primitive sentience" Gorovitz means the capacity to respond to sensory stimuli, then the transition from embryonic to fetal status (at the eighth week of gestation) or, at the latest, the tenth gestational week of fetal development would seem to mark the transition from nonprotected to protected status.[30] In fact, however, Gorovitz notes that he would draw the line of acceptability somewhat conservatively, that is, "rather close to the point where cell differentiation begins, rather far from the capacity for independent survival." [31]

A possible reason for the multiplicity of viewpoints on the status of the human embryo is suggested by Gorovitz. In his view, questions like embryonic status or the appropriate criteria of death are not matters of fact which can be clarified through appropriate research programs. Rather, these questions provide the occasion for individuals to make decisions and for societies to establish policies.[32] In contrast, while Kass does not directly address the fact/decision distinction, he clearly regards the discontinuity of fertilization and the continuity fo the embryonic development which follows as factual considerations which lead ineluctably to certain moral conclusions.[33]

E. *Potential Adverse Consequences of the Research.* Concerns about adverse consequences of laboratory research with human *in vitro* fertilization and embryo culture have been focused in three areas: (1) The same types of research *procedures* that have been performed with nonhuman mammalian embryos may be performed with human embryos; (2) certain undesirable technological or clinical *applications* may arise from such research; and (3) the research may have a desensitizing or dehumanizing *effect on investigators.*

Kass outlinés some of the scientific procedures which in his view are likely to be applied in the future to human embryos:

1. Culture beyond the blastocyst stage;
2. Formation of hybrids or chimeras (intra-specific and inter-specific);
3. Gene, chomosome, and plasmid insertion, excison, or alteration;
4. Nuclear transplantation or cloning; and
5. The freezing of embryos.[34]

Kass ventures this prediction because, in his view, the same arguments which can be advanced to justify, for example, the simpler and earlier procedures proposed by Pierre Soupart can without *logical* contradiction be extended to the more ambitious and later procedures outlined above. Among these justifiying principles are the following:

1. "It is desirable to learn as much as possible about the process of fertilization, growth, implantation, and differentiation of human embryos and about human gene expression and its control.
2. "It would be desirable to acquire improved techniques for enhancing conception and implantation, for *preventing* conception and implantation, for the treatment of genetic and chromosomal abnormalities, etc.
3. "Finally, only research using human embryos can answer these questions and provide these techniques.
4. "There should be no censorship or limitation of scientific inquiry or research."[35]

Without specifically advocating the types of experiments which Kass regards as undesirable, Gorovitz adopts a general position which could in principle allow him to approve such experiments. If one extrapolates from Gorovitz's views on embryonic status, one concludes that he would approve any type of research procedure on the human embryo, provided only that the research terminated prior to the onset of embryonic or fetal sentience and that other canons of research ethics (consent of gamete donors, appropriate research design, etc.)-were carefully followed.[36] Gorovitz explicitly accepts Kass's formal point that the justifying arguments for such research should be carefully formulated, in order to avoid the "slippery slope." [37] However, his material principle of drawing the dividing line at the point of sentience rather than fertilization or implantation seems, at least, to lead Gorovitz to approve as potentially beneficial the experiments which Kass regards as negative consequences of laboratory research with preimplantation embryos.

A specific research technique, interspecies fertilization using human sperm or ova, has provoked considerable discussion and therefore merits brief further comment. Cross-fertilization raises both conceptual and ethical questions. Conceptually, is fertilization research involving the use of only human sperm or human ova and the culture of the resultant hybrid embryo *human research?* Ethically, Kass regards such research as an adverse consequence of intraspecific *in vitro* fertilization. On the other hand, Short, while acknowledging that interspecific fertilization carries with it undertones of a novel type of genetic manipulation,[38] argues that technical and ethical hedges could be constructed to prevent what he regards as the major potential adverse consequence of such research—namely, any effort to transfer the hybrid embryo into the uterus of a human or animal female for further development.

A second type of potential adverse consequence identified by some critics of human *in vitro* fertilization and embryo culture concerns possible applications of the research rather than the research procedures themselves. Kass suggests that the research might lead to the banking of human ova or embryos for commercial purposes.[39] In the literature on this topic several other potential adverse consequences are noted: the cloning of human beings, the creation of human/animal hybrids, and the development of devices which would allow for the extracorporeal gestation, or ectogenesis, of human embryos and fetuses.[40] Without commenting specifically on these potential developments, Gorovitz expresses reservations about the wedge argument in its predictive (as distinguished from its logical) form. He also expresses confidence in the collective capacity of human beings to exercise good judgment, citing as examples public policy on abortion, appropriate treatment of newborn infants, the treatment of irretrievably comatose patients, and the setting of limits on the freedom of scientific inquiry.[41]

In an earlier essay on *in vitro* fertilization and cloning Leon Kass identified a third general type of potential adverse consequence which might result from laboratory research involving human embryos. According to Kass, one should "be concerned about the effects on the attitude toward and respect for human life engendered in persons who are engaged in such practices." [42] No other author has commented on the possibly dehumanizing effects on the researcher of human *in vitro* fertilization and embryo culture. It is probable that authors like Curran and Gorovitz would link the dehumanization question to the issue of embryonic or fetal status, arguing that only research on embryos which have developed beyond the two-to-three week stage (Curran) or to the point of sentience (Gorovitz) would show disrespect for the human embryo or fetus and that only research which manifested such disrespect would be likely to desensitize the researcher.

Footnotes

1. Short, R. V., Human *In Vitro* Fertilization and Embryo Transfer, a paper prepared for the Ethics Advisory Board, 1978, pp. 2–3; Mastroianni, Luigi, Jr., *In Vitro* Fertilization and Embryo Transfer, a paper prepared for the Ethics Advisory Board, 1978, p. 5.

2. Short, *op. cit.*, pp. 3–5; Mastroianni, *op. cit.*, p. 5.

3. Short, *op. cit.*, pp. 5–6.

4. Mastroianni, *op. cit.*, p. 5.

5. *Ibid.*

6. *Ibid.*

7. Short, *op. cit.*, pp. 6–7.

8. *Ibid.*, pp. 8–10.

9. Schlesselman, James J., How Does One Assess the risk of Abnormalities From Human *In Vitro* Fertilization?, a paper prepared for the Ethics Advisory Board, 1979, p. 17; cf. Biggers, John D., *In Vitro* Fertilization, Embryo Culture and Embryo Transfer in the Human, a paper prepared for the Ethics Advisory Board, 1978, p. 6 and Appendix I, Table 3.

10. Schlesselman, *op. cit.*, pp. 7–8, citing, Boue, J. G. and Boue, A., Chromosomal Anomalies in Early Spontaneous Abortion, *Current Topics in Pathology*, vol. 62, 1976, pp. 193–208; Creasy, M. R., Crolla, J. A., and Alberman, E. D., A Cytogenetic Study of Human Spontaneous Abortions Using Banding Techniques, *Humangenetik*, vol. 31, 1976, pp. 177–196, Alberman, E. D. and Creasy, M. R., Frequency of Chromosomal Abnormalities in Miscarriages and Perinatal Deaths, *Journal of Medical Genetics*, vol. 14, 1977, pp. 313–315.

11. Schlesselman, *op. cit.*, p. 19.
12. Short, *op. cit.*, p. 10; cf. Schlesselman, *op. cit.*, pp. 24–25.
13. Schlesselman, *op. cit.*, p. 30.
14. Biggers, *op. cit.*, p. 412; cf. Kass, Leon R., Ethical Issues in Human *In Vitro* Fertilization, Embryo Culture and Research, and Embryo Transfer, a paper prepared for the Ethics Advisory Board, 1978, p. 27.
15. Walters, LeRoy, Ethical Issues in Human *In Vitro* Fertilization and Research Involving Early Human Embryos, a paper prepared for the Ethics Advisory Board, 1978, fn. 178, citing Mastroianni, Luigi, Jr., *In Vitro* Fertilization, in: Reich, Warren, ed., *Encyclopedia of Bioethics*, (vol. 4), New York, Free Press-Macmillan, 1978, pp. 1448–1451.
16. Biggers, *op. cit.*, p. 41a.
17. Schlesselman, *op. cit.*, pp. 20–27.
18. Short, *op. cit.*, p. 9; cf. Walters, *op. cit.*, pp. 37–38.
19. Walters, *op. cit.*, fn. 182, citing National Research Council, Assembly of Behavioral and Social Sciences, Committee on the Life Sciences and Social Policy, *Assessing Biomedical Technologies: An Inquiry into the Nature of the Process*, Washington, D.C., National Academy of Sciences, 1975, p. 27.
20. *Ibid.*
21. Holder, Angela R. and Levine, Robert J., Informed Consent for Research on Specimens Obtained at Autopsy or Surgery: A Case Study in the Overprotection of Human Subjects, *Clinical Research*, vol. 24, 1976, pp. 68–77.
22. Kass, *op. cit.*, fn. 14, p. 28.
23. *Ibid.*, p. 5.
24. *Ibid.*, pp. 10–11.
25. *Ibid.*, p. 11.
26. Curran, Charles E., *In Vitro* Fertilization and Embryo Transfer: From a Perspective of Moral Theology, a paper prepared for the Ethics Advisory Board, 1978, p. 22.
27. *Ibid.*, p. 26.
28. Grobstein, Clifford, Statement to the Ethics Advisory Board, Transcript of Meeting III, September 15, 1978, *National Technical Information Service*, PB–288 764, p. 229.
29. Gorovitz, Samuel, *In Vitro* Fertilization: Sense and Nonsense, a paper prepared for The Ethics Advisory Board, 1979, p. 28.
30. Williams, John W., *Williams Obstetrics*, Pritchard, Jack A. and MacDonald, Paul C., eds., 14th ed., New York, Appleton-Century-Crofts, 1971, p. 223.
31. Gorovitz, *op. cit.*, p. 28.
32. *Ibid.*, pp. 1–4.
33. Kass, *op. cit.*, pp. 5–7.
34. *Ibid.*, pp. 18–19.
35. *Ibid.*, p. 20.
36. Gorovitz, *op. cit.*, pp. 27–28.
37. *Ibid.*, p. 15.
38. Short, *op. cit.*, p. 7.
39. Kass, *op. cit.*, p. 19.
40. Walters, *op. cit.*, pp. 39–40.
41. Gorovitz, *op. cit.*, p. 14.
42. Kass, Leon, Making Babies—the New Biology and the 'Old' Morality, *Public Interest*, vol. 26, 1972, p. 33.

Chapter III—Clinical Applications of in Vitro Fertilization and/or Embryo Transfer: Technical and Ethical Issues

A. The Need for and Potential Benefits of In Vitro Fertilization and Embryo Transfer

The major potential benefit to be derived from clinical applications of *in vitro* fertilization and embryo transfer is that it may enable some otherwise-infertile women to conceive and bear children. Most commentators on the clinical use of *in vitro* fertilization and embryo transfer view the alleviation of infertility, particularly in the context of heterosexual marriage, as a desirable goal.[1] In opposition to this majority position, however, Stanley Hauerwas argues that even within marriage, resort to *in vitro* fertilization as a method to overcome infertility reflects an undue emphasis on the importance of biological parentage.[2]

There are at least two senses in which the *need* for this potential benefit has been discussed. First, how many women who wish to bear children are infertile because of blocked Fallopian tubes? Second, of these infertile women, how many need *in vitro* fertilization and embryo transfer in the sense that they have no alternative means for producing children of their own?

Precise data on the extent of need in these two senses are unavailable. Rough estimates of the upper limits of need in the United States are provided by Biggers:

There are 60 million women reproductively active in the USA; seven percent of couples are infertile, and a third of these are infertile because of sterility of the wife. Thus, there are 1,400,000 sterile women in the population. Pathology of the oviduct accounts for 40 percent of the cases so that there are about 560,000 women with diseased oviducts.[3]

The major alternative to *in vitro* fertilization and embryo transfer for women is one of several surgical procedures available for repairing blocked oviducts: Salpingolysis, resection and reanastomosis, fimbrioplasty, and tubal implantation. According to a recent survey, the rates of term pregnancy following the first three of these procedures are 40-50%, 25–40%, and 10–25% respectively.[4] Thus, at least 280,000 U.S. women with tubal obstruction are not likely to achieve pregnancy by surgical methods alone. Of these women, an unknown number may also suffer from ovarian and/or uterine dysfunction and thus may be incapable of producing offspring even with the aid of *in vitro* fertilization and embryo transfer.[5] An additional adjustment in the estimate of the "need" for *in vitro* fertilization would be required if one were to consider women who had previously elected sterilization by tubal ligation but who later desire to become pregnant.

While the alleviation of infertility among couples is generally regarded as the major potential benefit of clinical *in vitro* fertilization and embryo transfer, some witnesses and some commentators in the literature have identified what they regard as additional benefits. Sid Leiman regards the surrogate-motherhood role as closely analogous to that of a wet nurse and therefore sees no ethical objection to extramarital involvement in gestation in cases in which intramarital reproduction is physically impossible.[6] In his writings on this topic R. G. Edwards mentions sex preselection as an additional potential benefit of clinical *in vitro* fertilization and embryo transfer.[7] Other potential benefits cited by various authors are pre-transfer screening for abnormalities,[8] re-transfer repair of defects,[9] and extracorporeal gestation.[10] The potential consequences enumerated in this paragraph are not universally judged to be beneficial, however, as Section F below illustrates.

B. The Need for and Adequacy of Prior Laboratory and Animal Research

Three major types of studies have been proposed as precursors to clinical applications of *in vitro* fertilization and embryo transfer: (1) Laboratory research on human sperm, ova, and embryos without embryo transfer, as described in Chapter 2, Section A above; (2) feasibility and safety studies in non-primate species; and (3) feasibility and safety studies in primates. Reservations have been expressed by some witnesses about each of these types of preliminary research.

Laboratory research with human sperm, ova, and embryos has been advocated most vigorously by R. V. Short. Short presents four arguments for a risk-assessment program based on such laboratory studies:

1. It would be better to discover an increased incidence, of abnormal embryos and/or low success rate "in the test tube rather than in the long-suffering female patient."

2. Laboratory tests could establish whether fertilization errors leading to potentially malignant trophoblastic tumors occur with *in vitro* fertilization.

3. Although chromosomally abnormal fetuses could be detected by amniocentesis, the discovery of such an affected fetus would confront an infertile couple with an agonizing decision; perhaps the decision would be viewed as a choice between having a handicapped child and no child at all.

4. Laboratory tests could establish whether

the lack of the natural screen against defective sperm which is provided by the female reproductive tract leads to an increase in the number of abnormal embryos produced *in vitro.*[11]

Four possible lines of objection to the type of risk-assessment study proposed by Short are suggested by the testimony of other witnesses. Biggers notes that large numbers of human ova would need to be collected and used in such studies in order to attain statistical significance and that the research would therefore involve a substantial number of women acting as donors.[12] Second, even if risk-assessment studies with human sperm, ova, and embryos were considered a necessary preliminary step, it can be argued that such studies would not be sufficient, since they would not detect the subtle types of mental or developmental deficits which might be discovered in a carefully conducted study of primates.[13] (As will be noted below, Short regards primate studies as too time-consuming.[14]) Third, in Biggers' view, there is already sufficient evidence from laboratory studies with rats, mice, and rabbits and from the use of embryo transfer in farm animals to justify the conclusion that *in vitro* fertilization and embryo transfer do not produce a significant increase in the number of abnormal offspring. On this view, the conduct of laboratory studies as proposed by Short is unnecessary.[15] A final type of objection to risk-assessment studies with human gametes and embryos can be derived from Schlesselman's essay—namely, that the efficiency of the human female reproductive system in screening against chromosomally abnormal embryos is so high (99.3% to 99.5%) that proceeding directly to embryo transfer in humans would probably not lead to a significantly higher number of abnormal fetuses (presumably detected by amniocentesis) or handicapped offspring. According to Schlesselman, the primary result of an increase in the number of embryonic chromosomal abnormalities would be an increased rate of spontaneous abortion.[16]

A second proposal is to perform feasibility and safety studies in non-primate species of laboratory animals, *e.g.*, the mouse and the rabbit. Mastroianni, a proponent of prior studies in both primate and non-primate species, asserts that:

> • • • Extensive work in the laboratory animal should be a necessary prerequisite before proceeding with clinical trials. Statistically valid proof in animals that present techniques predictably produce normal offspring has not as yet been presented. Successful uterine transfer of *in vitro* fertilized ova has been accomplished in only two laboratory species.[17]

Short's position is in part similar to that of Mastroianni. In his view, the results of research with laboratory animals "although somewhat inadequate, are on the whole encouraging. The high abnormality rate in the rat experiment [conducted by Toyoda and Chang [18]] was probably not due to the *in vitro* procedure at all (Chang, personal communication) but nevertheless the experiment should be repeated." [19]

Kass indicates his agreement with the "cautious" position of Luigi Mastroianni, Benjamin Brackett, and R. V. Short that:

> • • • The risks for humans have not been sufficiently assessed, in large part because the risks in animals have been so poorly assessed (due to the small number of such births and to the absence of any *prospective* study to identify and evaluate deviations from the norm).[20]

Two objections have been raised regarding studies with non-primate laboratory animals. First, Barton Childs observes that most animal species are so inbred that it would be invalid to extrapolate from the results of *in vitro* fertilization studies, even in large numbers of laboratory animals, to the probable result of clinical applications in humans, who are outbred.[21] Second, in Biggers' view the results of studies with various laboratory animals and of the use of the procedures in farm animals already provide sufficient evidence of safety.[22]

A third possible objection to further studies with non-primate animals is implicit in the Sackett proposal: subtle mental deficits caused by *in vitro* fertilization might not be detected in non-primate animals.[23] Fourth and finally, Schlesselman's calculations concerning the low probability of producing abnormal human offspring following *in vitro* fertilization and embryo transfer [24] can be viewed as an argument against performing further risk-assessment studies with laboratory animals.

A third proposal for preliminary risk-assessment studies is advanced by Sackett. He recommends the conduct of a two-year trial in the pigtail monkey which would include (1) *in vitro* fertilization with some embryos transferred back to the donors of the ova and some transferred to other females, (2) a study of the incidence of abnormalities in products of *in vitro* fertilization, and (3) an assessment of learning abilities and development in the offspring of *in vitro* fertilization.[25] Gould advocates the use of another primate model, the squirrel monkey, for risk-assessment studies.[26]

Several objections have been or can be lodged against the proposal to perform primate risk-assessment studies. Short comments on the time-investment required:

> Whilst it would be helpful to have primate data, the constraints inherent in studying this problem in primates mean that it would be several years before adequate information would be forthcoming, and it would seem wrong to hold up progress until the information was available.[27]

Childs echoes this objection.[28] Second, as noted above, Childs argues that all non-human species are relatively or strictly inbred, so that the range of genetic variability present in humans cannot be duplicated in non-human species.[29] Two other general objections are also applicable to proposed primate research: (1) The studies already performed in several non-primate species provide sufficient evidence concerning risks (Biggers [30]), and (2) abnormal human embryos resulting from *in vitro* techniques are likely to be spontaneously aborted (Schlesselman [31]).

In summary, there is a clear division of opinion within the scientific and ethical communities concerning the need for and adequacy of prior laboratory and animal research. The extent of the disagreement is unclear because not all of the expert witnesses have discussed the three alternative risk-assessment strategies outlined above. In particular, few experts have had the opportunity to comment specifically on the Short and Sackett proposals.

The following positions, however, have been stated with clarity. Biggers regards further risk-assessment studies of any kind as unnecessary. Childs, while acknowledging the reassurance that further animal studies might provide, argues that such studies could never provide conclusive evidence. Short, Mastroianni, Kass, Sackett, and Gould *agree* that further risk-assessment studies should be performed but *disagree* on what kind of studies would be most feasible and appropriate. Short advocates the performance of *in vitro* studies with human sperm and ova and the replication of a single rat study; he opposes primate studies on grounds of infeasibility and the amount of time required. Mastroianni and Kass support the performance of additional studies in animals, presumably in both primates and non-primates. Sackett and Gould regard non-primate risk-assessment studies as insufficient for drawing conclusions concerning primates and therefore recommend the conduct of primate research. In a word, there is majority support among the expert witnesses for some type of additional risk-assessment study but only minority support for any particular kind of study.

In addition, the data and calculations presented by Schlesselman may be relevant to the entire risk-assessment question. Schlesselman's thesis, which has not been commented on by proponents of risk-assessment studies, is that the probability of producing chromosomally-abnormal infants by means of clinical applications of *in vitro* fertilization and embryo transfer is quite low because of the human female's highly-efficient natural screen against chromosomally-abnormal embryos.

A little-discussed aspect of the risk-assessment debate is the kind of model (regarding proof of safety) which the protagonists have in mind. This model, in turn, can have important implications for the burden of proof issue. If one accepts the drug-testing model, as Short does, then the burden of proof is on investigators to demonstrate that the techniques of *in vitro* fertilization and embryo transfer are safe.[32] (It should be noted that, in a published essay, R. G. Edwards accepts the drug-tested model but argues that the results to date in several species of non-primate laboratory animals constitute sufficient proof of safety.[33]) On the other hand, if one adopts a surgery model, as Gorovitz does, than one can argue that the clinician is free to adopt new techniques unless opponents can demonstrate that prohibition of the techniques is justified.[34]

C. Risks of Procedures

1. Risks to Potential Offspring. The major sources of potential risk to offspring from *in vitro* fertilization and, embryo transfer have been briefly outlined in Chapter 1, Section B.[35] In general, the surgical procedure of embryo transfer seems to occasion the least concern, in part perhaps because of the widespread use of embryo transfer following natural fertilization in farm animals.[36] The conditions under which the early embryo is cultured are also not a matter of primary concern, since the early mammalian embryo is known to be highly resistant to damage from environmental insults.[37] The major potential sources of damage to the early embryo are related to either the development of ova, the selection of sperm, the fertilization process, or the freezing of gametes or embryos. Specifically, potential sources of damage are the following:

a. Superovulation, sometimes employed prior to *in vitro* fertilization, may be correlated with an increase in the incidence of a chromosomal abnormality (trisomy) in embryos.[38]

b. The quality of sperm reaching and fertilizing the ovum *in vitro* may differ from the quality of sperm fertilizing the ovum in the Fallopian tube, since the female reproductive tract selects against some types of abnormal sperm.[39]

c. The quantity of sperm reaching the ovum simultaneously *in vitro* may break down the usual block to fertilization by multiple sperm; a polyploid embryo may result.[40]

d. The use of freezing techniques to preserve gametes or embryos may produce mutations.[41]

The precise extent to which each of these theoretical sources of risk is likely to be realized in human clinical applications of *in vitro* fertilization and embryo transfer cannot be estimated with certainty. The data and calculations of Schlesselman suggest that even if an excess of chromosomally abnormal embryos were produced by *in vitro* techniques, only a small proportion (less than 10%) would develop to term because of the natural process by which most such embryos are lost early in gestation. Whether the ancillary medical treatment associated with *in vitro* fertilization and embryo transfer would enhance the survivability of chromosomally abnormal embryos is unknown, as Schlesselman acknowledges.[42] Similarly, if subtler genetic (as distinguished from chromosomal) abnormalities were to result from *in vitro* techniques, the abnormal embryos might not be affected by the natural screening process described by Schlesselman.

Judgments about the *acceptability* of various levels of risk to offspring diverge. Kass would require that such risks be equivalent to or less than those of natural reproduction.[43] Curran adopts a similar (although perhaps slightly less stringent) position, arguing that the risks of the *in vitro* fertilization and transfer procedures to the offspring ought to be "about the same as in the normal process."[44] On the other hand, Bigger notes that there is an estimated three percent additional risk of abnormality in offspring suggested by animal studies, and suggests that such an added risk would be acceptable, particularly in light of the fact that some couples who receive genetic counseling are not deterred from procreation by a twenty-five percent risk of genetically-abnormal offspring.[45]

Schlesselman explicitly raises the question: To what are the risks of human *in vitro* fertilization being compared? His answer is that the women and embryos being used for comparison should have the same medical history relevant to their infertility as those undergoing *in vitro* fertilization and embryo transfer.

2. Risks to donors. Most discussion of risks to donors has focused on risks to the women donating ova. The following sources of risk have been identified:

a. Hormonal treatment of the women, sometimes employed to induce superovulation; this treatment can lead to ovarian hyperstimulation or ovarian cysts.[46]

b. Laparoscopy, a surgical procedure generally performed under general anesthesia; this procedure may have to be repeated.[47]

c. Ectopic pregnancy, a potential danger if the embryo fails to implant in the uterus.[48]

d. Careful monitoring of any resulting uterine pregnancy, often including amniocentesis.[49]

e. The possibility of a higher-than-average rate of embryo loss or spontaneous abortion.[50]

These risks are considered to be comparable to the risks faced by female infertility patients, in general, and by women who undergo surgery for the correction of blocked Fallopian tubes, in particular.[51]

D. The Consent of Sperm and Ovum Donors

The issue of informed consent by sperm and oocyte donors was not addressed by the expert witnesses who testified before the Board. In the literature, however, there is unanimous agreement that the informed consent of the would-be mother and presumably of both parents must be secured. Several specific items of information have been identified by various commentators as being material to the decision of the couple and therefore requiring disclosure:

a. The availability of potentially effective alternative therapies, *e.g.*, surgical reconstruction of the Fallopian tubes.[52]

b. The anticipated need for repeated laparoscopies.

c. The low probability of success.

d. The likelihood that the primary beneficiaries of the research will be other couples rather than the research participants themselves.[53]

e. The sources of the gametes to be used in the attempted *in vitro* fertilization (*i.e.*, a guarantee that only the sperm and ova of the couple will be employed).[54]

f. The disposition to be made of sperm, ova, and embryos not used in the transfer attempt.[55]

In the literature on informed consent, several commentators have remarked that infertility patients may be strongly influenced by their desperate desire to have children.[56] On the other hand, R.G. Edwards notes that many candidates for *in vitro* fertilization and embryo transfer are professional persons or their wives. Edwards expresses confidence that the patients seeking this therapy are fully capable of understanding and consenting to its procedures.[57]

E. The Status of the Early Human Embryo

The question of embryonic status in the clinical context differs to some extent from the same question in the laboratory-research context. Perhaps the most obvious difference is that in the clinical context there is at least a possibility that each embryo "created" will be transferred to the uterus, will implant, and will develop to the point of viability. Because of this difference in probabilities, as well as the directly-therapeutic intention present in the clinical context, most expert witnesses on ethical issues surrounding *in vitro* fertilization and embryo transfer viewed the status of the early embryo as less problematic in the clinical situation.

For persons who regard the embryo as deserving of respect or protection from the time of fertilization there are two major concerns: (1) Loss of embryos following transfer, and (2) the disposition of untransferred embryos. Kass argues that there is no qualitative difference between embryonic loss following natural reproduction and that which follows *in vitro* fertilization.[58] The second issue is somewhat more complex, however, since, as Kass notes, the "surplus" embryos can be transferred to women other than the donor, used for laboratory research purposes, or allowed to die.[59] A fourth possibility, not mentioned by Kass, would be to freeze the untransferred embryos, perhaps for later transfer to the same donor. Among the first three possibilities, Kass expresses a clear preference for allowing untransferred embryos to die. In his view, this choice is most compatible with concerns about lineage (which would argue against transfer to other women) and about the respect which is owed to early human embryos.[60] Curran's position on the discard of embryos is similar to that of Kass, although Curran adds the note that discards and losses should be minimized insofar as possible.[61]

A potential method for reducing the number of untransferred embryos is suggested by both Kass and Leiman:[62] Ova could be fertilized one at a time, and any additional ova could be stored, perhaps by freezing, for future attempts at *in vitro* fertilization and embryo transfer. A possible objection to this one-at-a-time procedure is that if fertilization failed to occur, embryo transfer might be delayed until the next menstrual cycle.

An issue not discussed by the expert witnesses and only hinted at in the literaure on *in vitro* fertilization is the disposition of grossly abnormal embryos. Some have argued that to decide that such embryos should not be transferred is the first step toward deciding which fetuses (or persons) are not worthy to live.

Finally, some witnesses such as Gorovitz and Short do not explicitly consider the issue of embryonic status in the clinical context. However, if one extrapolates from their views on embryonic status in general or on laboratory research with early embryos, one can conclude with some confidence that they would regard the embryonic loss following embryo transfer and the discard of untransferred embryos as ethically acceptable.

F. Potential Adverse Consequences of Clinical Applications

Two types of potential adverse consequences of *in vitro* fertilization and embryo transfer have been identified: (1) Adverse consequences for the family; and (2) other adverse consequences. Kass notes that even if the initial aim of clinical applications is to assist married couples to bear children of their own, the techniques employed provide "the *immediate* possibility" of egg donation (egg from donor, sperm from husband), embryo donation (egg and sperm both from outside the marriage), and foster pregnancy (another woman carrying the pregnancy to term).[63] In Kass's view, there will be a strong demand for such extramarital uses of the clinical procedures—a demand which, if fulfilled, will further compromise "the virtues of family, lineage, and heterosexuality" or weaken "the taboos against adultery and even incest."[64]

Responses to the thesis that clinical uses of *in vitro* fertilization and embroyo transfer will weaken the family have taken two forms. The first, represented by Gorovitz, is to argue that the demand for labratory-assisted methods of reproduction in general will be limited and that other technological innovations (*e.g.*, modern contraceptive techniques) will have a much more significant adverse impact on the family.[65] A second kind of response, briefly developed by Leiman, is to deny that surrogate motherhood is necessarily detrimental to the family, if this novel method of becoming a parent is resorted to for good reasons (*e.g.*, if a couple would otherwise be unable to have a child).[66]

Other potential consequences considered adverse by some expert witnesses and commentators include:

a. The development of commercial ovum and embroyo banks.[67]
b. The genetic selection or manipulation of early embroyos.[68]
c. The transfer of nuclei from adult individuals to early embroyos, or cloning.[69]
d. Extracorporeal gestation, or bringing an embroyo all the way to viability in the laboratory.[70]

As noted in Section A of the present chapter, the second and fourth consequences in this list are regarded by some commentators as potential benefits of clinical *in vitro* fertilization and embryo transfer. Few have advocated that commercial ovum and embroyo banks be created or that human beings be cloned. Some commentators (for example, Gorovitz) have advanced the procedural suggestion that each potential consequence of *in vitro* fertilization and embryo transfer be carefully evaluated from the standpoint of both likelihood and probable impact.[71]

G. Questions of Allocation

Three general positions on the allocation issue can be distinguished. The first, represented by Biggers, is that applied laboratory research directed toward improving techniques for testing infertility by means of *in vitro* fertilization and embryo transfer should receive high priority—or, at least, that it should receive a higher priority than basic laboratory research involving human gametes and embroyos. The primary rationale for this position is Biggers' view that the supply of human ova available for research purposes is extremely limited and should devoted either to directly clinical purposes or to answering questions that cannot be satisfactorily resolved by studying laboratory animal.[72]

A second position, represented by Leiman[73] and Curran,[74] is that the federal government should support the clinical application of *in vitro* fertilization and embyro transfer. Leiman regards involuntary infertility as an extremely serious problem.

> The rabbis put it this way, some fifteen centuries ago. Four are considered as if they were dead: the poor, the diseased, the blind, and the childless.[75]

In his view, the public funding of medical means for overcoming infertility (for example, through Medicaid) is entirely appropriate. Indeed, Leiman argues that:

> It would be a sad commentary on the American ethos if federal funds could be

used for the taking of human life, that is, therapeutic abortion, but not the creation of human life, that is, therapeutic conception.[76]

Although Kass disagrees with this second position; he presents an additional argument which some have used to support it:

> * * * As he who pays the piper calls the tune, Federal support would make easy the Federal regulation and supervision of this research.[77]

In contrast, a third position on allocation is that Federal funds should not be spent for *in vitro* fertilization and embryo transfer in clinical practice. Hauerwas, Gorovitz, and Kass all take this position, although for somewhat different reasons. In Hauerwas' view, the importance of being pregnant or of bearing a child that is genetically "one's own" has been overstated. Therefore the substantial investment of public funds to develop these anti-infertility techniques, particularly in light of other "immense needs of our society," (for example, the provision of an effective clotting factor for hemophiliacs) is inappropriate.[78] While he may not share Hauerwas' views on parenthood, Gorovitz agrees with his sense of priorities.

> In the competition for support, the burden of making a convincing case should rest with the proponent of a given line of work. With forty million Americans having no adequate access to decent health care, with thousands of children born annually without prospect of a family to nurture them, with veneral disease—a major cause of infertility—on the rise, it is implausible that research into making IVF more readily and reliably available should be a project of high priority concern. It isn't so much the harm or risk it involves as the plainly greater importance of addressing more fundamental and widespread problems of health and the delivery of health care.[79]

Kass presents three arguments for assigning a low priority to clinical applications of *in vitro* fertilization and embryo transfer. First, in agreement with Hauerwas and Gorovitz, he asserts that other health-related needs are more pressing. Kass goes on to argue that even within the sphere of infertility research, other approaches will be more cost-effective:

> * * * With money for research as limited it is, research funds targeted for the relief of infertility should certainly go first to epidemiological and preventive measure—especially where the costs of success in the high-technology cure are likely to be *great.*[80]

Second, according to Kass, the non-financial costs of developing these technologies—that is, their potential adverse consequences—also militate against assigning their development a high priority.[81] Finally, Kass notes that a substantial number of American citizens are opposed on moral grounds to research on, or application of, *in vitro* fertilization in humans. In his view, these citizens would strenuously—and legitimately—object to any use of their taxes to promote human *in vitro* fertilization and embryo transfer.[82]

Footnotes

1. Kass, Leon R., Ethical Issues in Human *In Vitro* Fertilization, Embryo Culture and Research, and Embryo Transfer, a paper prepared for the Ethics Advisory Board, 1978, pp. 13–14; Leiman, Sid Z., Statement to the Ethics Advisory Board, Transcript of Meeting V, November 10, 1978 *National Technical Information Service*, PB–288 405, p. 130.
2. Hauerwas, Stanley, Theological Reflections on *In Vitro* Fertilization, a paper prepared for the Ethics Advisory Board, 1978, pp. 6–12.
3. Biggers, John D., *In Vitro* Fertilization, Embryo Culture and Embryo Transfer in the Human, a paper prepared for the Ethics Advisory Board, 1978, p. 35.
4. Biggers, *op. cit.*, p. 36 and Table 4, p. 37, citing Shane, J. M., Schiff, I., and Wilson, E. A., The Infertile Couple, *Clinical Symposia*, vol. 28, 1976, pp. 1–40.
5. Biggers, *op. cit.*, p. 35; Kass, *op. cit.*, pp. 36–37.
6. Leiman, *op. cit.*, pp. 126–130.
7. Walters, LeRoy, Ethical Issues in Human

In Vitro Fertilization and Research Involving Early Human Embryos, a paper prepared for the Ethics Advisory Board, 1978, fn. 112, citing Edwards, R. G., Fertilization of Human Eggs *In Vitro:* Morals, Ethics, and the Law, *Quarterly Review of Biology*, vol. 49, 1974, p. 12.

8. Walters, *op. cit.*, fn. 113, citing Karp, Laurence E. and Donahue, Roger P., Preimplantational Ectogenesis: Science and Speculation Concerning *In Vitro* Fertilization and Related Procedures, *Western Journal of Medicine*, vol. 124, 1976, p. 295.

9. Walters, *op. cit.*, fn. 115, citing Sinshiemer, Robert L., Prospects for Future Scientific Developments: Ambush or Opportunity, in: Hilton, Bruce *et al.*, eds., *Ethical Issues in Human Genetics: Genetic Couseling and the Use of Genetic Knowledge*, New York, Plenum Press, 1973, pp. 346–348.

10. Walters, *op. cit.*, fn. 118, citing Fletcher, Joseph, *The Ethics of Genetic Control: Ending Reproductive Roulette*, Garden City, N.Y., Anchor Press/Doubleday, 1974, pp. 163–165.

11. Short, R. V., Human *In Vitro* Fertilization and Embryo Transfer, a paper prepared for the Ethics Advisory Board, 1978, p. 9.

12. Biggers, John D., Statement to the Ethics Advisory Board, Transcript of Meeting III, September 16, 1978, *National Technical Information Service* PB–288 764, pp. 235–239.

13. Sackett, Gene P., A Nonhuman Primate Model of Developmental Risk Following *In Vitro* Fertilization and Embryo Transfer, a paper prepared for the Ethics Advisory Board, 1979, pp. 26–28.

14. Short, *op. cit.*, p. 8.

15. Biggers, Statement to the Ethics Advisory Board, *op. cit.*, pp. 257, 260–261.

16. Schlesselman, James J., How Does One Assess the Risk of Abnormalities from Human *In Vitro* Fertilization?, a paper prepared for the Ethics Advisory Board, 1979, pp. 29–31.

17. Mastroianni, Luigi, Jr., *In Vitro* Fertilization and Embryo Transfer, a paper prepard for the Ethics Advisory Board, 1978 p. 6.

18. Toyoda, Y. and Chang, M. C., Fertilization of Rat Eggs *In Vitro* by Epididymal Sperm and the Development of Eggs Following Transfer, *Journal of Reproduction and Feritlity*, vol. 36, 1976, pp 9–22.

19. Short, *op. cit.*, p. 8.

20. Kass, *op. cit.*, 1978, pp. 12–13.

21. Childs, Barton, Statement to the Ethics Advisory Board, Transcript of Meeting III, September 16, 1978, *National Technical Information Service*, PB–288 764, pp. 252–253.

22. Biggers, Statement to the Ethics Advisory Board, *op. cit.*, pp. 257, 260–261.

23. Sackett, *op. cit.*, pp. 26–28.

24. Schlesselman, *op. cit.*, pp. 29–31.

25. Sackett, *op. cit.*, pp. 31–32.

26. Gould, Kenneth G., Fertilization *In Vitro* of Nonhuman Primate Ova: Present Status and Rationale for Further Development of the Technique, a paper prepared for the Ethics Advisory Board, 1978, pp. 21–23.

27. Short, *op. cit.*, p. 8.

28. Childs, *op. cit.*, p. 232a.

29. *Ibid.*

30. Biggers, Statement to the Ethics Advisory Board, *op. cit.*, pp. 257, 260–261.

31. Schlesselman, *op. cit.*, pp. 29–31.

32. Short, *op. cit.*, pp. 8–10.

33. Walters, *op. cit.*, fn. 50, citing Edwards, R. G., Fertilization of Human Eggs *In Vitro:* Morals, Ethics and the Law, *Quarterly Review of Biology*, vol. 49, 1974, pp. 8–9.

34. Gorovitz, Samuel, *In Vitro* Fertilization: Sense and Nonsense, a paper prepared for the Ethics Advisory Board, 1979, p. 24.

35. See Chapter I of this report, pp. 9–10.

36. Short, *op. cit.*, p. 8; Foote, R. H., *In Vitro* Fertilization in Perspective, Relative to the Science and Art of Domestic Animal Reproduction, a paper prepared for the Ethics Advisory Board, 1978, p. 17.

37. Biggers, *op. cit.*, p. 34.

38. Biggers, *op. cit.*, p. 34, citing Boue, J. G. and Boue, A., Increased Frequency of Chromosomal Anomalies in Abortions After Induced Ovulation, *Lancet*, vol. i, 1973, p. 679.

39. Biggers, *op. cit.*, p. 33, citing Ahlgren, M., Sperm Transport to and Survival in the Human Fallopian Tube, *Gynecologic Investigation*, vol. 6, 1975, pp. 206–214.

40. Biggers, *op. cit.*, p. 33, citing Fraser, L. R., Zenellotti, H. M., Paton, G. R. and Drury, L. M., Increased Incidence of Triploidy in Embryos Derived from Mouse Eggs Fertilized *In Vitro*, *Nature*, vol. 260, 1976, pp. 39–40; Fraser, L. R., and Maudlin, I., Relationship Between Sperm Concentration and the Incidence of Polyspermy in Mouse Embryos Fertilized *In Vitro*, *Journal of Reproduction and Fertility*, vol. 52, 1978, pp. 103–106.

41. Biggers, *op. cit.*, p. 34.
42. Schlesselman, *op. cit.*, pp. 29–31.
43. Kass, *op. cit.*, 1978, p. 12.
44. Curran, Charles E., *In Vitro* Fertilization and Embryo Transfer: From a Persepective of Moral Theology, a paper prepared for the Ethics Advisory Board, 1978, p. 19.
45. Biggers, Statement to the Ethics Advisory Board, *op. cit.*, pp. 261–263; see also Shulman Joseph, Testimony for the Ethics Advisory Board, 1978, p. 3.
46. Gould, *op. cit.*, p. 17; Mastroianni, *op. cit.*, p. 3.
47. Gould, *op. cit.*, pp. 17–18.
48. *Ibid.*, pp. 18–19.
49. *Ibid.*, p. 19.
50. Schlesselman, *op. cit.*, pp. 29–31.
51. Gould, *op. cit.*, p. 17; Edwards, *op. cit.*, p. 8; Mastroianni, Luigi, Jr., *In Vitro* Fertilization, in: Reich, Warren, ed., *Encyclopedia of Bioethics*, vol. 4, New York, Free Press-Macmillan, 1978, pp. 1448–1451.
52. Kass, Leon, Making Babies—the New Biology and the Old' Morality, *Public Interest*, vol. 26, 1972, p. 31.
53. Items (b) through (d) are enumerated in: National Research Council, Assembly of Behavioral and Social Sciences, Committee on the Life Sciences and Social Policy, *Assessing Biomedical Technologies: An Inquiry into the Nature of the Process*, Washington, D.C., National Academy of Sciences, 1975, p. 21.
54. British Medical Association, Board of Science and Education Panel, *Professional Standards*, London, British Medical Association, 1972, p. 10.
55. National Research Council, *op. cit.*, pp. 21, 27.
56. Mastroianni, Luigi, Jr., *In Vitro* Fertilization of Human Ova and Blastocyst Transfer: An Invitational Symposium, in: Schumacher, Gebhard, F., *et al.*, *Journal of Reproductive Medicine*, vol. 11, 1973, p. 197; National Research Council, *op. cit.*, 1975, p. 21.
57. Edwards, *op. cit.*, p. 11.
58. Kass, *op. cit.*, pp. 9–10.
59. *Ibid.*, p. 10.
60. *Ibid.*, pp. 9–11.
61. Curran, *op. cit.*, pp. 17, 26.
62. Kass, *op. cit.*, 1972, p. 34; Leiman, *op. cit.*, p. 126.
63. Kass, *op. cit.*, 1978, p. 15.
64. *Ibid.*
65. Gorovitz, *op. cit.*, pp. 20–21.
66. Leiman, *op. cit.*, pp. 128–129.
67. Kass, *op. cit.*, 1978, p. 19.
68. Walters, *op. cit.*, fn. 113 (see fn. 9 above).
69. *Ibid.*
70. *Ibid.*, fn. 118 (see fn. 10 above).
71. Gorovitz, *op. cit.*, pp. 14–15.
72. Biggers, Statement to the Ethics Advisory Board, *op. cit.*, pp. 236–237.
73. Leiman, *op. cit.*, pp. 130–131.
74. Curran, *op. cit.*, p. 28.
75. Leiman, *op. cit.*, p. 131.
76. *Ibid.*
77. Kass, *op. cit.*, 1978, p. 22.
78. Hauerwas, *op. cit.*, p. 18.
79. Gorovitz, *op. cit.*, p. 26.
80. Kass, *op. cit.*, 1978, p. 25.
81. *Ibid.*
82. *Ibid.*, pp. 28–29.

Chapter IV—Legal Issues Surrounding Human in Vitro Fertilization, Embryo Culture, and Embryo Transfer

Two papers written for the Board examined the legal issues surrounding human *in vitro* fertilization; one was prepared by Dennis Flannery and his colleaques at the Washington law firm of Wilmer, Cutler and Pickering, the other was written by Barbara Katz, Office of Legal Affairs, University of Colorado Medical Center. The discussion which follows reflects the legal analysis and conclusions presented by the two papers; in any areas where they differed, the differences are noted. Four main topics are addressed: (A) Existing law that might be applicable to human *in vitro* fertilization and embryo transfer; (B) Constitutional questions raised either by the use, or by restrictions imposed on the use, of the techniques; (C) possible implications for tort liability; and (D) criminal law.

A. Existing Federal and State Law Applicable to Human in Vitro Fertilization and/or Embryo Transfer

1. *Federal law.* The only existing federal control of human *in vitro* fertilization is a regulation of the Department of Health, Education, and Welfare:

> No application or proposal involving human *in vitro* fertilization may be funded by the Department or any component thereof until the application or proposal has been reviewed by the Ethical Advisory Board and the Board has rendered advice as to its acceptability from an ethical standpoint.[1]

In its notice of proposed rulemaking entitled "Protection of Human Subjects: Proposed Policy" issued August 23, 1974, the Department indicated the kind of issues it expected the Ethics Advisory Board to consider:

> With respect to the fertilization of human ova *in vitro*, it is expected that the Board will consider the extent to which current technology permits the continued development of such ova, as well as the legal and ethical issues surrounding the initiation and disposition of such products of research.
>
> With respect to implantation of fertilized human ova, it is expected that the Board will consider such factors as the safety of the technique (with respect to offspring) as demonstrated in animal studies and clarification of the legal responsibilities of the donor and recipient parent(s) as well as the research personnel.[2]

Two other general requirements of HEW regulations are presumably applicable to research involving human *in vitro* fertilization, as well. All such research conducted or supported by the Department must be reviewed by a local Institutional Review Board (IRB);[3] in addition, studies involving human *in vitro* fertilization should not be conducted or supported by HEW unless "appropriate studies on animals and nonpregnant individuals have been completed."[4]

Moreover, the Department interprets the National Research Act as authorizing (if not requiring) IRB review of human research not funded by HEW at any institution which receives a grant or contract involving human subjects under the Public Health Service Act.

> The Secretary shall by regulation require that each entity which applies for a grant or contract under this Act for any project or program which involves the conduct of biomedical or behavioral research involving human subjects submit in or with its application for such grant or contract assurances satisfactory to the Secretary that it has established (in accordance with regulations which the Secretary shall prescribe) a board (to be known as an 'Institutional Review Board') to review biomedical and behavioral research involving human subjects conducted at or sponsored by such entity in order to protect the rights of the human subjects of such research.[5]

However, the standards to be employed by the local Institutional Review Board in reviewing non-federally funded human research are not specified by the statute.

2. *State law.* No state has enacted legislation or promulgated regulations directly governing human *in vitro* fertilization and/or embryo transfer. Such laws or regulations could affect the conduct of research involving *in vitro* fertilization within particular jurisdictions, especially since the federal regulations governing such research specifically do not preempt state or local law in this sphere:

> Nothing in this subpart shall be construed as indicating that compliance with the procedures set forth herein will in any way render inapplicable pertinent State or local laws bearing upon activities covered by this subpart.[6]

The types of existing law which provide the closest analogies to human *in vitro* fertilization and/or embryo transfer are state statutes or court decisions concerning (a) artificial insemination and (b) research involving human fetuses.

Within the context of family law, the issue of artificial insemination, especially artificial insemination with donor sperm (AID), has received legislative or judicial attention in approximately one-third of the states. Case law concerning AID has focused primary attention on whether AID is equivalent to adultery and thus, whether children conceived as a result of AID are legitimate. (Legitimacy has implications both for inheritance rights and for claims to paternal support.) The general trend of recent case law, particularly in California and New York, has been toward the view that AID does not constitute adultery and that children conceived as a result of AID are legitimate.[7] Nineteen states have enacted legislation regarding one or more aspects of artificial insemination; many of the statutes include a requirement for prior written consent by both husband and wife.[8] However, in the remaining states, the legal status of children conceived following AID is left in doubt.

A second area of state legislative interest—research with live human fetuses—is also at least partially analogous to research involving human *in vitro* fertilization. Approximately sixteen states have enacted statutes governing fetal research. The primary focus of all such statutes is the permissibility of research on the fetus (1) following implantation and (2) before, during, or after induced abortion. however, the language of at least one state statute on fetal research may be sufficiently broad to encompass, as well, research involving unimplanted early human embryos.[9]

B. Constitutional Issues

1. *Preliminary Distinctions.* Federal or state action may be found unconstitutional if it infringes upon a fundamental right of United States citizens and the government cannot demonstrate (1) that the law is necessary to protect a "compelling state interest" and (2) that it does not go beyond what is necessary to protect those interests.[10] If, on the other hand, a governmental action restricts individual activities in ways that do not infringe a fundamental right, then the government need only show that its action is rationally related to a constitutionally permissible purpose.[11] Thus, a critical question regarding human *in vitro* fertilization—whether in the laboratory or the clinical context—will be whether individuals proposing to employ, or seeking access to, the technique can be said to be asserting a fundamental legal right. This, in turn, determines whether the government will be required to justify its regulation of human *in vitro* fertilization by demonstrating a compelling state interest that it seeks to protect or only by demonstrating a rational basis for its action.

A second distinction is also important: the distinction between a governmental restriction of an activity, on the one hand, and a governmental decision not to fund the activity, on the other. In 1977, in a case challenging the constitutionality of restrictions on the use of Medicaid funds for abortions, the United States Supreme Court held that a governmental restriction of the use of public funds to support the exercise of a fundamental right does not, by itself, constitute impermissible interference with the exercise of that right.[12] The Court concluded that the existence of a fundamental right "implies no limitation on the authority of a state to make a value judgment [to discourage the exercise of that right] and to implement that judgment by the allocation of public funds." [13] As applied to the question of *in vitro* fertilization, that language suggests that a governmental decision to restrict either laboratory research or clinical applications of the technique would need stronger justification than would a decision not to provide funds for such activities.

2. *Clinical Applications of In Vitro Fertilization and Embryo Transfer.* Constitutional principles affecting reproductive activity are more fully articulated than those relating to basic laboratory research. Therefore, it is useful to examine the rights pertaining to reproductive choices before attempting to analyze what rights might be implicated in government regulation

of basic laboratory research.

The argument for a constitutional right to reproduce by means of *in vitro* fertilization would rest on the right to privacy as related to procreation, the marital relationship, and contraception. In 1942, in a decision striking down Oklahoma's compulsory sterilization law, the Supreme Court held that individuals have a right to be free from unwarranted governmental interference with procreative capabilities. (*Skinner* v. *Oklahoma*) [14] This might be termed "the right to procreation." [15] A second constitutionally protected area is the privacy of the marital relationship. This was recognized in a 1965 decision (*Griswold* v. *Connecticut*) invalidating a Connecticut statute forbidding the use of contraceptives by married couples. There, the Court said:

> The entire fabric of the Constitution and the purposes that clearly underlie its specific guarantees demonstrate that the rights to marital privacy and to marry and raise a family are of similar order and magnitude as the fundamental rights specifically protected . . . . The fact that no particular provision of the Constitution explicitly forbids the State from disrupting the traditional relation of the family—a relation as old and as fundamental as our entire civilization—surely does not show that the Government was meant to have the power to do so.[16]

The privacy interests recognized in Griswold were expanded in later cases to include "the right of the individual, married or single, to be free from governmental intrusion into matters so fundamentally affecting a person as the decision whether to bear or beget children." [17]

The extent to which any individual's access to *in vitro* fertilization will be viewed as involving a fundametal right will depend upon how closely analogous it is to the rights recognized by the Supreme Court. Thus, for example, a married couple with no alternative means for having a child of their own could claim that restriction of access to *in vitro* fertilization is interference with the fundamental right of marital privacy and with their right to choose whether, and in what manner, to achieve procreation. Since these rights are reasonably analogous to those recognized by the Court in *Skinner, Griswold,* and *Eisenstadt,* the argument might well be persuasive. If the Court agreed with the view that the rights in this instance are fundamental, the government would have to demonstrate a compelling state interest to justify interfering with the exercise of those rights.

On the other hand, an unmarried woman who wished to utilize *in vitro* fertilization followed by embryo transfer to another (sorrogate) mother, in order to have a genetic child of her own without the expense and inconvenience of pregnancy, would have a much weaker case. There would be neither marital privacy nor a procreative capacity, in the normal sense, to protect. Thus, courts might well find the right asserted to be less than fundamental, and the government would have to show only a rational basis for restricting the exercise of that "right".

Several grounds for prohibiting or limiting access to clinical applications of *in vitro* fertilization could be advanced. First, a state or the federal government might argue that this reproductive technique inevitably involves the loss of human embryos. Accordingly, a government might enact legislation to protect early human embryos. Such a law might pass the rational basis test but might not withstand constitutional challenge by individuals who could assert a fundamental right to access to *in vitro* fertilization.[18]

A second possible basis for state intervention in the clinical applications of *in vitro* fertilization would be the government's interest in fostering marriage and discouraging illegitimacy. This rationale might be proffered, for example, in support of a law restricting publicly funded *in vitro* fertilization and emryo transfer to married couples.[19] This is little room for doubt that such a funding limitation would be found constitutionaly permissable; it is not clear, however, whether courts would uphold an outright prohibition on the access of single persons to *in vitro* fertilization and embryo transfer.[20]

Third, a government might prohibit or limit access to clinical applications of *in vitro* fertilization in order to preclude institutional or individual genetic planning or manipulation. It is been suggested that the potential social impact of a large-scale genetic program might justify governmental regulation, but that interference with the genetic planning of individual families would have to be justified by a compelling state interest.[21]

Fourth, a state or the federal government might conclude that the use of surrogate or host mothers in connection with clinical *in vitro* fertilization would create insuperable legal problems that would justify a prohibition of such activities—perhaps on the ground that service as a surrogate mother is an unacceptable form of employment.[22] In the opinion of Flannery and associates such a prohibition would probably withstand legal challenge on both "rational basis" and "compelling state interest" grounds.[23]

Finally, if clinical applications of *in vitro* fertilization should appear to present health risks to mother or offspring which are substantially greater than those usually associated with conception and childbirth, then a state or the federal government might well decide to prohibit or limit access to this reproductive technique. Whether such a state intervention would withstand constitutional challenge would depend in part on the probability and magnitude of the risks involved.[24]

In addition to making basic decisions regarding the regulation of access to clinical applications of *in vitro* fertilization, the states and the federal government may wish to establish policies on such related matters as the legal status of children who are produced by means of *in vitro* fertilization and embyro transfer, the role of attending physicians in decisions regarding implantation and abortion, and record-keeping requirements.[25]

3. *Laboratory Research Involving In Vitro Fertilization and/or Embryo Culture*—a. *Constitutional bases for asserting a right to perform or participate in laboratory research involving in vitro fertilization and/or embyro culture.* Two major constitutional arguments could be advanced in support of basic laboratory research involving human *in vitro* fertilization. The first is freedom of inquiry, or the right of scientists to perform their research without governmental interference. This argument can be asserted most vigorously in defense of research conducted without the assistance of government funding. The second is the right of individual's to dispose of their genetic material as they see fit.

In a recent report, the National Commission for the Protection of Human Subjects of Biomedical and Behavorial Research expressed the view that although the Supreme Court might recognize a First Amendment right to seek new ideas or knowledge (i.e., a "right to research")[26], that must be distinguished from a right to be free from regulations governing the manner in which research may be conducted.[27]

> * * * [T]he state may not interfere with the researcher's choice of the end or topic of research, but it may regulate only the methods used in the research, in order to protect interests in health, order and safety with which unrestricted research might conflict. Such restrictions are valid if they are reasonably related to protection of non-speech interests and are not so vague and

over broad that they chill the exercise of protected speech.[28]

Accepting the National Commission's distinction between the goal and the manner of research as valid, then the applicability of this putative right to basic research involving human *in vitro* fertilization is problematic, since it is the manner of achieving the knowledge—that is, through the creation and study of human embryos—that is most likely to be the target of governmental regulation.[29]

A second constitutional argument in support of laboratory research involving human *in vitro* fertilization focuses attention on the rights of potential gamete donors to dispose of their reproductive cells in whatever manner they see fit. According to this view, donors have a "constitutionally protected fundamental privacy right to control the use and manipulation of their own genetic materials.[30] Such a privacy right is clearer, however, in cases involving contraception or abortion than in the case of genetic materials donated for basic laboratory research. Once the materials are outside the body of the donor, any personal rights of privacy regarding their use become attenuated.[31]

b. *Constitutional bases for governments' prohibiting or refusing to fund laboratory research involving human in vitro fertilization.* If the analysis of the preceding section is accepted, than it would appear that no fundamental constitutional right to perform or participate in basic research involving *in vitro* fertilization is likely to be found. In the absence of such a right, the government could, if it wished, prohibit *in vitro* fertilization research if it had a rational basis for doing so. A prohibition would most probably be based on the view that the creation, study, and destruction of early human embryos is inconsistent with the dignity which should be accorded to forms of potential human life. Even if a fundamental right to conduct or participate in such research did exist, the government could still decline to support it with public funds. Such a refusal could be based on an administrative determination that other areas of research would be more useful to the government.[32]

If research with early human embryos were to involve embryo transfer and subsequent implantation, the current HEW regulations governing fetal research would apply, since the "fetus" is defined as the embryo "from the time of implantation."[33] State statutes regarding fetal research might or might not apply, depending on their formulation.

In addition to deciding whether to prohibit or to support laboratory research involving human *in vitro* fertilization, states or the federal government might wish to formulate standards governing the conduct of such research, if the research is permitted. For example, regulations to protect the health of ovum donors or to set standards for protecting the dignity of potential human life might be adopted. Moreover, a government might require that gamete donors consent in advance to the use of their reproductive cells in research involving *in vitro* fertilization. These procedural regulations, designed to achieve a rational governmental purpose, should be constitutionally permissible.[34]

C. Liability for Injuries

The federal government might be liable for injuries arising from *in vitro* fertilization in research programs conducted or supported by HEW. This section explores three questions: (1) Whether such suits would be barred by the doctrine of sovereign immunity; (2) what causes of action might be considered valid; and (3) whether a program could be established to provide compensation for such injuries.

1. *Sovereign immunity.* Under the Federal Tort Claims Act, the United States is liable for the "negligent or wrongful" acts or omissions of its employees while they are acting within the scope of their employment.[35] Exceptions to such liability include acts or omissions that are within an agency or officer's "discretionary duty" (as, for example, a decision to initiate a particular research program).[36] Whether the doctrine of sovereign immunity would bar a suit for damages arising within an HEW-conducted or supported research program involving *in vitro* fertilization would depend upon:

1. Whether the investigator is considered a federal "employee." (Does this category include, for example, grantees or contractors in HEW-funded research programs?)
2. Whether the alleged wrong occurred because of the employee's exercise of protected "discretionary functions" at the policy level or through a failure to exercise due care in a particular program at the operational level.
3. Whether the employee's act fell within an exception to liability under the Federal Tort Claims Act.

The Board's legal consultants suggest that the United States, but not individual investigators, would probably be liable for any negligence of subordinate HEW officers or employees who design or conduct a particular research program involving in vitro fertilization. If the conduct violated existing HEW regulations, even the discretionary exception would not prevent liability.[37]

2. *Possible causes of action*—a. *Actions on behalf of the child.* Two kinds of suits might be brought on behalf of a child born alive with handicaps following *in vitro* fertilization and embryo transfer. First, a suit might be brought on the basis of prenatal or even preconception injuries sustained by the child. (Preconception injuries might be claimed if, for example, laboratory procedures involving the gametes were thought to have given rise to the damage.) The plaintiff in such a suit would face the difficult task of demonstrating a causal connection between the procedures of *in vitro* fertilization or embryo transfer and the child's injuries.[38]

Alternatively, a "wrongful life" suit might be brought on behalf of a child born alive but handicapped following *in vitro* fertilization and embryo transfer. Such a suit would claim that it would be better for a child not to be born at all than to be born in a damaged condition. With one exception,[39] the courts have refused to recognize "wrongful life" as a valid ground for recovery of damages. This refusal appears to stem from a reluctance or inability to assign a monetary value to either impaired existence or nonexistence as a basis for recovery.[40] Even if "wrongful life" were accepted as a valid cause of action in principle, the plaintiff would still face the challenge of showing a causal connection between the procedures employed and the child's injuries.[41]

b. *Actions to compensate the parents.* Two distinct types of suit might be brought under this general heading. First, it might be claimed that negligently-caused damage to a child conceived by means of *in vitro* fertilization had caused the parents economic loss and/or emotional distress. Courts have held that the following "wrongful birth" suits stated a valid cause of action:

1. The mother of a severely deformed child brought suit against her physician for his failure to diagnose rubella during pregnancy.[42]
2. Parents brought suit against a physician for failing to diagnose a pregnancy in time to allow the woman to secure an abortion.[43]
3. A pharmacist was sued for mistakenly filling a prescription for the contraceptive Norinyl with a different drug, Nardil, when the woman subsequently became pregnant.[44]
4. A couple brought suit against a physician whose sterilization of the husband failed to prevent the wife's conception of a subsequent child.[45]

If a "wrongful birth" suit were brought

because of the birth of a handicapped child following *in vitro* fertilization, the plaintiff would face the difficulties of demonstrating causation which have been alluded to in the preceding paragraphs.[46]

A second possible cause of action which might be brought by would-be parents on their own behalf is an action for the "wrongful death" of a hoped-for child. All states currently allow actions for wrongful death caused by prenatal injuries if the death occurs following live birth. In addition, many states allow recovery for the prenatal death of a viable fetus.[47] The question raised by *in vitro* fertilization and embryo transfer is whether the theory of "wrongful death" would be extended by the courts to cover preimplantation human embryos.

Under a somewhat different legal theory—one which focused on the destruction of the would-be parents' property rather than on the "wrongful death" of an early embryo—a New York jury recently awarded $50,000 for emotional distress following the intentional destruction of a culture containing gametes from the husband and wife.[48] In the opinion of Flannery and associates, it is unlikely that the courts will ultimately extend the concept of "wrongful death" to include the intentional destruction of a preimplantation embryo.[49] According to Katz, suits charging physician negligence in the unintentional death of an embryo or fetus conceived with the aid of *in vitro* fertilization are also unlikely to succeed because of the experimental character of the procedure and because of the absence of a clear standard of due care.[50]

3. *Compensation for injury.* In part because traditional tort concepts seem inapplicable to research involving *in vitro* fertilization and/or embryo transfer, Katz proposes the establishment of a federal compensation fund to provide monetary redress in the event of injury associated with such research.[51] In her view, the rationale for creation of such a fund is that society has a substantial interest in establishing a program of human *in vitro* fertilization research and therefore has an obligation to the human subjects who may be injured as a result of their participation in such a program. Any injury which is not clearly unrelated to participation in the *in vitro* fertilization program would be compensable. The amount of compensation would be determined by calculating the monetary requirements for making the situation of a damaged child or mother equal to that of a normal person, insofar as such calculation is possible. The compensation fund would be financed through premiums paid by researchers or their institutions, by adding a surcharge to hospital bills, or by allocating general revenues to this purpose. The plan would include financial incentives to encourage the exercise of due care by investigators and institutions.

D. Criminal Law

The primary question of criminal law that might arise is whether the act of allowing preimplantation human embryos to die or killing them would constitute the crime of feticide, a species of homicide. After surveying developments in English and American jurisprudence, Katz concludes that the destruction of preimplantation human embryos is not likely to fall within either homicide or feticide statutes.[52]

As noted above, however, state statutes enacted to regulate research involving human fetuses may be broad enough to include research involving preimplantation human embryos. For example, one state statute defines the "human conceptus" as "any human organism, conceived either in the human body, or produced in an artificial environment other than the human body, from fertilization through the first 265 days thereafter."[53]

The statute continues:

> Whoever uses or permits the use of a living human conceptus for any type of scientific, laboratory research or other experimentation except to protect the life or health of the conceptus, or except as herein provided, shall be guilty of a gross misdemeanor.[54]

In summary, aside from HEW regulations governing research supported by the Department, and a very few broadly written state statutes prohibiting research on the human fetus, no state or federal laws apply to human *in vitro* fertilization. However, Supreme Court decisions recognizing a fundamental right to privacy in marital relations and reproductive activity suggest that married couples might successfully assert a right of access to *in vitro* fertilization and embryo transfer as a means of bearing their own children. The government would have to demonstrate a compelling state interest (*e.g.*, protecting the health and safety of mothers and offspring) to justify restricting such access. The government need not, however, provide federal support for such procedures. In the research context, the government may regulate the manner in which research is conducted, especially if the research is supported by funds and it involves human subjects. Questions about legal responsibility for the care of the offspring cannot be answered with clarity. Analogous statutory and case law in the field of artificial insemination suggests that the law in this area is confused, at best. Similarly, questions about liability and compensation for injuries to the mothers and offspring need to be addressed.

Footnotes

Note.—The two papers prepared for the Board and cited often throughout are: Dennis M. Flannery, *et al.*, "Legal Issues Concerning *In Vitro* Fertilization" (hereinafter cited as, Flannery *et al.*) and Barbara F. Katz, "Legal Implications of *In Vitro* Fertilization and Its Regulation" (hereinafter cited as Katz).

1. 45 CFR § 46.204(d).
2. 39 Federal Register 30650, August 23, 1974.
3. 45 CFR § 46.205.
4. 45 CFR § 46.202(a)(1).
5. Public Law 93–348, 88 Stat. 348, July 12, 1974.
6. 45 CFR § 46.201(b).
7. Katz, pp. 6–10; cf. Flannery *et al.*, pp. 48–49.
8. Katz, pp. 6–10; cf. Flannery *et al.*, pp. 48–49.
9. Flannery *et al.*, pp. 5–6; Katz, pp. 42–44.
10. Flannery *et al.*, p. 35.
11. Maher v. Roe, 432 U.S. 464, 478 (1977).
12. Flannery *et al.*, p. 35.
13. Maher v. Roe, 432 U.S. 464, 474 (1977).
14. Skinner v. Oklahoma, 316 U.S. 535 (1942).
15. Flannery *et al.*, p. 10.
16. Griswold v. Connecticut, 381 U.S. 479 (1965).
17. Eisenstadt v. Baird, 405 U.S. 438, 453 (1972); *see also*, Carey v. Population Services International 431 U.S. 678 (1977).
18. Flannery *et al.*, pp. 38–40; Katz, p. 49.
19. Flannery *et al.*, p. 40.
20. *Id.* at 41–42.
21. *Id.* at 42–44.
22. *Id.* at 45, n. 68.
23. *Id.* at 45–46.
24. *Id.* at 46–47; Katz, p. 49.
25. Flannery *et al.*, pp. 47–54.
26. National Commission for the Protection of Human Subjects of Biomedical and Behavioral Research. *Institutional Review Boards: Report and Recommendations,* DHEW Publication No. (OS) 78–0008, U.S. Government Printing Office, Washington, D.C., 1978, p. 78. (Discussed in Flannery *et al.*, p. 58 *et seq.*)
27. *Id.* at 79.
28. *Id.*
29. Flannery *et al.*, p. 60; Katz, pp. 45–46.
30. Flannery *et al.*, p. 61.
31. *Id.* pp. 61–63; Katz, p. 49.
32. Flannery *et al.*, pp. 63–65.
33. 45 CFR § 46.203(d).
34. Flannery *et al.*, pp. 70–72.
35. 28 U.S.C. § 1346(b); Flannery *et al.*, pp. 73–74.
36. 28 U.S.C. § 2680(a).
37. Flannery *et al.*, pp. 76–82.
38. Katz, p. 15; Flannery *et al.*, pp. 85–86.
39. Park v. Chessin, 60 App. Div.2d 80, 400 N.Y.S.2d 110 (1978).
40. Katz, p. 18; Flannery *et al.*, p. 87.

41. Katz, p. 18.
42. Jacobs v. Theimer, 519 S.W.2d 846 (Texas 1975); cited by Katz, pp. 18–19.
43. Ziemoa v. Sternberg, 400 N.Y.2d 110 (1977); cited by Katz, p. 19.
44. Troppi v. Scarf, 187 N.W.2d 511 (Mich. 1971); cited by Katz, p. 19 and Flannery *et al.*, p. 88.
45. Doerr v. Villate, 220 N.E.2d 767 (Ill. 1966); cited by Katz, p. 19.
46. Katz, pp. 19–20; Flannery *et al.*, pp. 88–89.
47. Flannery *et al.*, p. 88; Katz, pp. 29–30.
48. Del Zio v. Presbyterian Hospital, 1974 Civ. 3588 (S.D.N.Y. 1978).
49. Flannery *et al.*, p. 88.
50. Katz, p. 27.
51. Katz, pp. 32–37.
52. Katz, pp. 21–25.
53. Minn. Stat. Ann. § 145.521, section 2 (West 1977); cited by Flannery *et al.*, n. 19.
54. Minn. Stat. Ann. § 145.522, (West 1977); cited by Flannery *et al.*, n. 19.

Chapter V.—Review of Public Attitudes

A. Responses Received by the EAB

Between September 15 and December 15, 1978, the Ethics Advisory Board held eleven public hearings on the question of federal support of research involving human *in vitro* fertilization (IVF) in order to afford an opportunity for members of the public to present their views. In all, several thousand hearing notices were sent to professional organizations, public interest groups, universities, clergy, and individuals. Everyone who requested to appear was heard; 179 individuals presented testimony in hearings in Bethesda (Maryland), Boston, Seattle, San Francisco, Atlanta, Kansas City, Detroit, Philadelphia, Denver, Dallas and New York City. Eighteen people preferred to submit formal written testimony in lieu of oral presentation. In addition, the Board received over 2000 letters and postcards, some of which were forwarded from President Carter and Secretary Califano.

Transcripts of all formal presentations (both oral and written) have been distributed to members of the Board and are available to the general public from the National Technical Information Service (NTIS). All of the correspondence received by the Board has been duplicated and distributed to members; copies are on file at the office of the EAB and are available for public inspection.

In the arguments and presentations made to the Board, it was evident that many people did not distinguish between basic research involving laboratory fertilization of human ova (IVF) on the one hand, and the subsequent transfer of the resulting embryos to establish a pregnancy, on the other. Thus, some of the arguments both for an against "*in vitro* fertilization" referred only to one or another of the procedures under consideration by the Board. At the public hearings, it was often possible to elicit clarification by asking whether a person's statement was intended to apply to both the basic research and the clinical application; this was not the case with respect to written communications. Summaries of the arguments are presented below.

1. *Arguments in favor of Federal Funding.* Although there were, of course, many variations on the theme, most of the arguments in favor of federal support of IVF focused on either the risks and benefits of IVF or the rights of investigators and infertile couples: (a) The scientific benefits to be gained; (b) the need for federal regulation; (c) the necessity to evaluate and to reduce the risks inherent in the procedure and the reliance of such research on federal suppport; (d) freedom of inquiry for scientists; (e) freedom of reproductive choice for infertile couples; and (f) the rights of infertile couples to some return on their taxes paid for general health and welfare.

The majority of individuals who favor federal funding for research involving human IVF stressed the benefits it would produce for the general welfare (*e.g.*, understanding and correcting infertility, preventing birth defects, understanding certain hereditary diseases, furthering the search for a cure for cancer, improving our knowledge of early fetal development, and developing better methods of contraception). A number of witnesses stated that there are many scientific procedures that can be used for either the benefit or the detriment of mankind; but the possibility for abuse does not in and of itself make their development morally wrong. Many responded to the concern regarding "discards" by noting that fertilized eggs are often lost in the natural process of reproduction. Some stated that it is morally irrelevant whether embryo loss occurs naturally or in a laboratory. Other individuals pointed out that zygote wastage may eventually be eliminated. For example, it may be possible to extract only one ovum at a time, as suggested by Dr. Steptoe (on Meet the Press), once the techniques of fertilization and embryo transfer are improved. Moreover, some public witnesses stated that once the technique of freezing the embryos is perfected, fertilized eggs that are not transferred immediately may be preserved for later attempts at implantation.

Numerous witnesses expressed concern about the possible risks of embryo transfer procedures already being performed in the private sector. A few stressed the need to hold investigators accountable for their actions; others urged federal support of the activities in order to apply regulations to assure that they will be conducted in a responsible manner. They thought that if the government were to fund research and adopt regulations governing the experimentation, investigators receiving non-government money would follow the government regulations.

Some stressed the need for government support to assure greater exploration of animal models and to encourage basic research in human IVF so that the safety and efficacy of the procedure can be evaluated before clinical application of embryo transfer is permitted. A related argument was that if research is permitted, scientists may be expected to improve the technique of *in vitro* fertilization and embryo transfer so that risks to mother and offspring will be substantially reduced.

Several individuals stressed the responsibility of the government to assure freedom of inquiry. Others urged the government to educate the public about the significance of new scientific discoveries to the public. They were concerned that the development of federal policy with such profound implications might be influenced by a public unnecessarily alarmed by inaccuracies and misinterpretations.

The last set of arguments in favor of federal funding related to the rights of infertile couples as taxpayers and the corresponding duties of the government. A number of individuals felt that since childless couples have paid taxes that subsidize the costs of contraception and childbearing, as well as education and welfare, for other people's children, the government has an obligation to assist them by supporting research and services relevant to their reproductive needs. Some argued that it is the government's responsibility to ensure freedom of choice for women by making both alternatives—raising a family or remaining childless—available to all couples.

It was stated that at the present time, adoption is not a viable alternative for childless couples. The waiting list for infants is very long and the cost for international adoption is exhorbitant and limited. There was additional testimony, however, that even if adoption procedures could be improved, problems would remain; adoption does not satisfy the very strong desire to bear one's own child. Some even suggested that the unfulfilled desire to bear children threatens the mental health of women and the stability of marriages. They argued that infertility is a disorder requiring medical intervention, and that the government has a responsibility to make such health care available to all citizens. Since the government funds therapeutic abortions when bearing a child would threaten the life or health of the mother, they noted, the government ought to fund "therapeutic conception" as well. Some elaborated on this argument, stating that government funding is necessary to assure that the option of having a child through *in vitro* fertilization is available to poor women as well as to those who are able to purchase the option in the private sector.

2. *Arguments Opposed to Federal Funding.* In general, the arguments against federal support of IVF and embryo transfer stemmed from five major concerns: (a) The moral status of the embryo; (b) questions of safety; (c) funding priorities; (d) decreasing ability to limit more objectionable procedures; and (e) detrimental social and psychological effects on offspring, family and physicians.

The most frequently articulated argument against federal funding of IVF was based on the moral status of the fertilized egg and embryo. Proponents of this argument believed that human life should be respected from the moment of fertilization. They argued that deliberately to create human life merely for experimental purposes with no intent or expectation of sustaining such life is immoral.

Since many fertilized eggs are discarded in the normal process of procreation some proponents of this position said that they might not oppose *in vitro* fertilization research if a technique could be perfected that would allow the investigators to extract and fertilize only one egg, or freeze for later transfer the embryos which could not be implanted immediately. Others stated that even if such a technique were perfected, it would still be unethical to fund *in vitro* fertilization research because of the immorality of interfering with the natural process of human reproduction.

Many individuals expressed concern about proceeding with embryo transfer in humans without further data concerning its safety. They believed that more should be known about the probability of producing defective embryos. They also thought it important to gain more information concerning level of risk to the women undergoing the procedures. Among opponents of federal funding on the grounds of safety were those who thought that people have a right to take risks by volunteering for research conducted in the private sector, but that it is unethical for the government to approve and support IVF and embryo transfer in humans before the risks and benefits have been more fully evaluated.

A large number of persons opposed government funding of IVF and embryo transfer because they believe it is not an important national priority. Various other needs were suggested as having greater claims upon government funds. A favorite alternative was research to develop methods of preventing and treating disorders (such as pelvic infectious diseases) that result in the tubal occlusion giving rise to demands for IVF. Others indicated that funds would be better spent in improving fertility control and in learning to prevent or treat birth defects and genetic abnormalities. Still others stressed society's responsibility toward those children already in existence who have been abused or abandoned. Programs encouraging adoption should have higher priority than IVF. There were also those who believed it **inappropriate to fund IVF when the majority, they were certain, opposed** such research on deeply-felt ethical or religious grounds. The government should not spend public money for experiments so clearly in conflict with the basic commitments of many of the citizens.

Some expressed a fear that approving policies that permit researchers consciously to intend human life to die *in vitro* could lead to an inability to draw barriers to policies that allowed more obviously objectionable occasions for humans to end the life of other humans. Some proponents of this argument believed that the selective destruction of undesirable fertilized eggs might contribute to the creation of a eugenic program controlled by some officially condoned elite. There was even the fear that barriers would fall to the creation of half-animal, half-human hybrids or chimeras.

A variety of harmful consequences to the psychological and social well-being of those involved in IVF were cited as reasons for not funding such research. Fears were expressed that children born through *in vitro* fertilization would initially be subject to considerable notoriety and be unable to escape a continuing stigma. There was concern that IVF might endanger the family by reducing the human act of reproduction to an artificial or mechanical laboratory procedure. An even greater threat to the family would be the possible use of surrogate mothers and extra-marital donors of genetic material. This set of reasons for opposing government funding of IVF included the dehumanizing of scientists and doctors involved in the research who must dispose of the human embryos. Another possible consequence cited as a reason for opposing funding was the possible exploitation of uneducated, poor and minority women.

B. *Public Opinion Surveys*

Since the birth of Louise Brown on July 25, 1978, both the Gallup and Harris survey organizations have conducted polls providing the clearest indication available of United States public opinion concerning IVF. The Gallup survey included reactions of both men and women. The Harris survey, conducted August, 1978 for *Parents* magazine, polled 1,501 representatively selected American women. Both polls revealed that majority opinion favors IVF. However, most women in the Harris survey wanted IVF prohibited until further testing had established its safety, and they opposed federal funding of research on IVF.

Gallup reported that 60% of both men and women "favored" the operation. Of persons who could fully explain the procedure, 75% approved, indicating that more knowledge of IVF led to greater acceptance. Approval was even higher among the women in the Harris poll. Eighty-five percent said that the procedure should be an option for couples otherwise unable to have children.

As to whether Americans would be willing to avail themselves of the operation, the two polls reported that a majority would do so. Gallup found 53% of Americans generally would undergo the procedure. Harris reported that 58% of women of childbearing age would consider using IVF. More specifically defined groups among childbearing women produced even more favorable attitudes: 61% of younger women, age 18–39, approved of IVF, as did 66% of the women actually planning to have children.

While most women in the Harris survey approved of IVF as a legitimate option, when they were asked if they couldn't have children would they prefer adoption or IVF, more than twice as many chose adoption (57%) as IVF (21%). Furthermore, a healthy majority (63%) wanted IVF to be banned as standard medical practice until further research had determined whether the operation increased the likelihood of birth defects. (Only 24% wanted IVF available immediately.) Interestingly, although most women wanted further testing of IVF, half (50%) opposed federal funding of such research.

Chapter VI—Summary and Conclusions

It is now technically possible to fertilize a human egg outside the body of a woman and then transfer the fertilized egg (sometimes called a blastocyst or preimplantation embryo) back into the woman to establish a pregnancy. For some women, *in vitro* fertilization may be the only way to bear children of their own. It does not appear, however, that the procedure for achieving pregnancy by this means is yet very effective; the best available data indicate that a number of attempts have been necessary before a pregnancy in a particular woman can be established, if at all. In addition, many questions remain as to the safety of the procedure for the offspring. Nevertheless, there is reason to believe that clinics may soon be established, both in this country and abroad, where *in vitro* fertilization and embryo transfer will be offered as "therapy" for infertile couples.

The Board is required by HEW regulations to review research proposals involving human *in vitro* fertilization and advise the Secretary as to their "acceptability from an ethical standpoint." [1] This phrase is broad enough to include at least two interpretations: (1) "Clearly ethically right" or (2) "ethically defensible but still legitimately controverted." In finding that research involving human *in vitro* fertilization is "acceptable from an ethical standpoint" the Board is using the phrase in the second sense; the Board wishes to emphasize that it is *not* finding that the ethical considerations against such research are insubstantial. Indeed, concerns regarding the moral status of the embryo and the potential long-range consequences of this research were among the most difficult that confronted the Board.

In its deliberations on human *in vitro* fertilization, the Board confronted many ethical, scientific and legal issues. Among the more difficult were the following: (A) The moral status of the embryo; (B) the safety and efficacy [2] of the procedure; (C) the potential long-range adverse effects of such research; and (D) the appropriateness of Departmental support.

A. After much analysis and discussion regarding both scientific data and the moral status of the embryo, the Board is in agreement that the human embryo is entitled to profound respect; but this respect does not necessarily encompass the full legal and moral rights attributed to persons. In addition, the board noted the high rate of embryo loss that occurs in the natural process of reproduction. It concluded that some embryo loss associated with attempts to assist otherwise infertile couples to bear children of their own through *in vitro* fertilization be regarded as acceptable from an ethical standpoint, under certain conditions, as more fully described below.

B. The Board is concerned about still unanswered questions of safety for both mother and offspring of *in vitro* fertilization and embryo transfer; it is concerned, as well, about the physical and mental health of the children born following such a procedure and about their legal status. Many women have told the Board that in order to bear a child of their own they will submit to whatever risks are involved. The Board believes that while the Department should not interfere with such reproductive decisions, it has a legitmate interest in developing and disseminating information regarding

[1] 45 CFR 46.204(d).

[2] By "efficacy" the Board means not only whether the procedure can be done but also how efficient it is, *e.g.*, the number of procedures required to achieve the desired result.

safety and health so that fully informed choices about reproduction can be made.

C. A number of fears have been expressed with regard to adverse effects of technological intervention in the reproductive process: fears that such intervention might lead to genetic manipulation or encourage casual experimentation with human embryos, or bring with it the use of surrogate mothers, cloning, or the creation of genetic hybrids. Some have suggested that such research might also have a dehumanizing effect on investigators, the families involved, and society generally. (See Chapter III of this report.)

Although the Board recognizes that there is an opportunity for abuse in the application of this technology as other technologies, it concluded that a broad prohibition of research involving human *in vitro* fertilization is neither justified nor wise. Among the developments warned against by some who testified before the Board, a few (*e.g.*, the cloning of human beings and the creation of animal/human hybrids) are of uncertain or remote risk. Other possible developments, such as the use of surrogate mothers, may be contained by regulation or legislation. Other abuses may be avoided by the use of good judgment based upon accurate information of the type collected by the Board and now being disseminated in this report. Finally, where reproductive decisions are concerned, it is important to guard against unwarranted governmental intrusion into personal and marital privacy.

D. The question of Federal support of research involving human *in vitro* fertilization and embryo transfer was troublesome for the Board in view of the uncertain risks, the dangers of abuse and because funding the procedure is morally objectionable to many. In weighing these considerations, the Board noted that the procedures may soon be in use in the private sector and that Departmental involvement might help to resolve questions of risk and avoid abuse by encouraging well-designed research by qualified scientists. Such involvement might also help to shape the use of the procedures through regulation and by example. The Board concluded that it should not advise the Department on the level of Federal support, if any, of such research; but it concluded that Federal support, if decided upon after due consideration of all that is at issue, would be acceptable from an ethical standpoint.

Evidence presented to the Board indicates that human *in vitro* fertilization and embryo transfer techniques may, in the near future, be employed throughout the world in both research and clinical practice settings. The Board believes that data from these activities as well as related types of animal research should be collected, analyzed and, when appropriate, given wide public dissemination. Accordingly, the Board recommends in conclusion #4 below, that the Department take the primary initiative in carrying out these functions.

Having carefully weighed diverse ethical points of view and a broad base of scientific considerations regarding human *in vitro* fertilization and embryo transfer, the Board has concluded that: (1) The Department should consider support of more animal research in order to assess the risks to both mother and offspring associated with the procedures; (2) the conduct of research involving human *in vitro* fertilization designed to establish the safety and effectiveness of the procedures is ethically acceptable under certain conditions; (3) Departmental support of such research would be acceptable from an ethical standpoint, although the Board did not address the question of the level of funding, if any, which such research might be given; (4) the Department should take the initiative in collecting, analzing and disseminating data from both research and clinical practice involving *in vitro* fertilization throughout the world; and (5) model or uniform laws should be developed to define the rights and responsibilities of all parties involved in such activities.

Finally, the Board is aware of the possibility of research that involves the collection and culture of early human embryos in the laboratory which have been fetilized naturally rather than *in vitro*. The ethical aspects of such research, which appears to bear a close resemblance to research involving *in vitro* fertilization, have not been examined by the Board. Therefore it has not reached a conclusion concerning the ethical acceptability of these procedures. However, the Board intends to consider in the near future the need for setting standards for such research.

Conclusion (1).—The department should consider support of carefully designed research involving *in vitro* fertilization and embryo transfer in animals, including nonhuman primates, in order to obtain a better understanding of the process of fertilization, implantation and embryo development, to assess the risks to both mother and offspring associated with such procedures, and to improve the efficacy of the procedure.

Discussion: As indicated in Chapter III of the Board's report, available scientific data do not indicate clearly either the relative safety or the efficacy of procedures of *in vitro* fertilization and embryo transfer. Some scientists have suggested that *in vitro* fertilization may result in a higher incidence of abnormal embryos than is associated with the normal reproductive process, although there are no animal data that clearly demonstrate such an effect. Neither are there data that demonstrate an absence of increased abnormality in embryos following *in vitro* fertilization. The Board feels that additional data should be gathered that might indicate whether abnormal embryos are more likely to result and, if so, whether there is a significant increase in the risk of abnormal offspring actually being born following such procedures.

Experts appearing before the Board agreed that there has been insufficient controlled animal research designed to determine the long-range effects of *in vitro* fertilization and embryo transfer. The lack of primate work is particularly noteworthy in view of the opportunity provided by primate models for assessing subtle neurological, cognitive and developmental effects of such procedures. The Board has been advised that controlled studies of embryo transfer following *in vitro* fertilization in animals, designed to include developmental assessments, may be feasible and may permit more confident estimates of the risk to human offspring associated with such procedures.

Information regarding the effectiveness of the procedures for *in vitro* fertilization and embryo transfer is also lacking. It does not appear possible to predict with reliability the number of laparoscopies and embryo transfers that might be required, or the likelihood of success of the procedure for any couple, given the fact that, to date, only three successes have been reported in humans, and that very limited information is available concerning this work. Such data as are available suggest that any woman hoping to bear a child through *in vitro* fertilization is likely to face numerous unsuccessful procedures and delays with no assurance of achieving her goal.

Careful research with animal models might provide a more accurate estimate of the chances of achieving a successful pregnancy. It might also reduce the inconvenience and risk to women of undergoing multiple procedures to establish a pregnancy by improving techniques for recovering ova, identifying embryonic abnormalities and achieving implantation. It is often the case in medicine that, even after therapies are already being applied to humans, investigations continue in animals in order to test further or to improve their safety and effectiveness. The Board believes that the Department should consider support of well-designed animal studies whether or not human research or clinical trials are also in progress.

Conclusion (2)—The ethics advisory board finds that it is acceptable from an ethical standpoint to undertake research involving human *in vitro* fertilization and embryo transfer provided that:

A. If the research involves human *in vitro* fertilization without embryo transfer, the following conditions are satisfied:

1. The research complies with all appropriate provisions of the regulations governing research with human subjects (45 CFR 46);

2. The Research is designed primarily: (A) To establish the safety and efficacy of embryo transfer and (B) to obtain important scientific information toward that end not reasonably attainable by other means;

3. Human gametes used in such research will be obtained exclusively from persons who have been informed of the nature and purpose of the research in which such materials will be used and have specifically consented to such use;

4. No embryos will be sustained *in vitro* beyond the stage normally associated with the completion of implantation (14 days after fertilization); and

5. All interested parties and the general public will be advised if evidence begins to show that the procedure entails risks of abnormal offspring higher than those associated with natural human reproduction.

B. In addition, if the research involves embryo transfer following human *in vitro* fertilization, embryo transfer will be attempted only with gametes obtained from lawfully married couples.

Discussion: This conclusion relates to the ethics of conducting research involving *in vitro* fertilization in general; it does not address the question of Departmental support of such research. The purpose of this more general conclusion is to provide guidance to Institutional Review Boards and other groups who are asked to review research that will not be supported by HEW.[3] Whether or not the Department decides to provide funds for such research, the Board wishes to express its views regarding the conduct of human *in vitro* fertilization and embryo transfer, so that review groups may benefit from the deliberations of the Board as they conduct their own review of specific research proposals.

As emphasized above, the Board believes that much remains to be learned about the safety and effectiveness of these procedures before they can be considered standard, accepted medical practice. Research designed to provide reliable data regarding safety and efficacy is acceptable from an ethical standpoint if conducted within the constraints indicated above. In the case of research involving embryo transfer, the Board intends not only that the gametes be obtained from lawfully married couples but also that the embryo be transferred back to the wife whose ova were used for fertilization.

The Board also discussed research designed primarily to establish safety and efficacy but which may, in addition, obtain information of scientific importance unrelated to *in vitro* fertilization and embryo transfer. The

[3] Federal law requires all institutions receiving research funds from HEW to establish an Institutional Review Board (IRB) to review biomedical and behavioral research involving human subjects. (Pub. L. 93-348). The Department, in implementing that law, requires all such research conducted at an institution to be reviewed by the IRB, whether or not the research is supported by HEW.

Board believes that such research, if performed as a corollary to research designed primarily to establish safety and efficacy of *in vitro* fertilization and embryo transfer, would also be acceptable from an ethical standpoint.

Conclusion (3)—The Board finds it acceptable from an ethical standpoint for the department to support or conduct research involving human *in vitro* fertilization and embryo transfer, provided that the applicable conditions set forth in conclusion (2) are met. However, the Board has decided not to address the question of the level of funding, if any, which such research might be given.

Discussion: 1. *Departmental support.* The Board consciously adopted the language "acceptable from an ethical standpoint" to indicate the limits of its inquiry. Even though the members are aware that ethical considerations pervade decisions regarding the level, if any, of Departmental support of human *in vitro* fertilization, the Board has concluded that it lacks the resources needed to render meaningful advice with respect to such decisions. The Board, therefore, defers to established political, scientific and administrative procedures for allocating public research funds.

The Board wishes to note that such decisions have significant ethical dimensions. For example, some believe that research involving human *in vitro* fertilization should have a relatively low priority at a time when other health needs, arguably more basic in character and long-term in nature, are unmet. Others find such research objectionable either on grounds related to the moral status of the embryo or because it may lead to undesirable genetic interventions or have a long-range adverse effect. (See Chapter III of this report.) Still others believe that research on human *in vitro* fertilization and embryo transfer should have a high priority because it might help parents overcome physical obstacles to having their own children and ensure the mothers' safety and the normality of offspring.

The Board has found that these and other ethical arguments for and against public funding of research involving human *in vitro* fertilization, by themselves, are not conclusive. Instead, the Board believes that the questions of whether to fund and at what level should be made in the larger context where all relevant data and arguments—scientific, political, economic, legal and ethical—can be considered. In that context questions such as health and safety, availability of funds, and alternative research proposals, must be considered along with the very difficult type of ethical issues described above which arise in allocation of resources.

2. *Research without embryo transfer.* As previously noted the risks of producing abnoraml offspring are still undertermined; therefore, an important goal would be to gain as much information as possible from well-designed research on *in vitro* fertilization not involving embryo transfer in humans. The Department should conduct a careful scientific evaluation of the possibility, supported by some expert testimony before the Board, that animal research and studies involving human *in vitro* fertilization without embryo transfer, over a relatively short period, might substantially increase our knowledge concerning the possible risk of abnormal offspring as well as lead to the development of safe and more effective techniques.

3. *Research involving embryo transfer.* While initial research efforts designed to gain as much information as possible form animal studies and human research not involving embryo transfer may be desirable, the Board does not wish to discourage planning and preparation that may lead to clinical trials or other forms of research

involving embryo transfer. The Department's participation in, or support of, clinical trials is often an effective method to evaluate the safety and efficacy of innovative medical procedures, particularly as the use of the procedures increases.

4. *Research for other purposes.* Potentially valuable information about reproductive biology, the etiology of birth defects, and other subjects may be revealed through research involving human *in vitro* fertilization without embryo transfer, and unrelated to the safety and efficacy of procedures for overcoming infertility. The Board makes no judgment at this time regarding the ethical acceptability of such research nor does it speculate about what research might be sufficiently compelling to justify the use of human embryos. Instead, it notes that applications for support of such research should be submitted to the Board for ethical review in accordance with 45 CFR 46.204(d).

5. *Pending Research Application.* Given the criteria specified in Conclusion (2) and incorporated in Conclusion (3) for evaluating research involving human *in vitro* fertilization, and the Board's views about Departmental support of such research, the Board recommends that the Secretary refer the pending application of Vanderbilt University back to the National Institutes of Health for a determination as to whether the proposal meets those criteria and for further review in light of the considerations set forth in this report.

Conclusion (4)—The national institute of child health and human development (NICHD) and other appropriate agencies should work with professional societies, foreign governments and international organizations to collect, analyze and disseminate information derived from research (in both animals and humans) and clinical experience throughout the world involving *in vitro* fertilization and embryo transfer.

Discussion: The Board is aware that the most valuable information regarding *in vitro* fertilization and embryo transfer is likely to come from well-controlled clincial trials. But it is expected that *in vitro* fertilization and embryo transfer will soon be performed in clinics throughout the world, sometimes without benefit of research design or experimental controls. It would be unfortunate not to have access to the information that might be gained from such clinical experience, notwithstanding the fact that well-designed investigations would be preferable. With that in mind, the Board recommends that every effort be made to collect whatever information may be elicited from practitioners in this country and abroad. NICHD should also consider suggesting to practitioners a basic protocol for collecting vital information, to which each would be encouraged to add their own observations.

The data from such clinical experience and from research conducted throughout the world should be analyzed along with that derived from animal studies so that individuals contemplating *in vitro* fertilization and embryo transfer will have access to the best information available regarding risks to both mother and offspring. Timely dissemination of the information would increase the opportunity for investigators, clinicians and prospective patients to be fully informed.

Conclusion (5)—The secretary should encourage the development of a uniform or model law to clarify the legal status of children born as a result of *in vitro* fertilization and embryo transfer. To the extent that funds may be necessary to develop such legislation, the department should consider providing appropriate support.

Discussion: The Board is concerned about the ambiguity regarding the legal status of children born following artificial insemination and a similar ambiguity that may surround the legal status of children born following *in vitro* fertilization and embryo transfer. The Board is also concerned about lack of clarity regarding the legal responsibilities of those who utilize, support, or permit use of such procedures. Because of the complexity of the legal problems involved in new techniques for human reproduction, the Board recommends that a model or uniform law be drafted that would establish with clarity the rights and responsibilities of donor and recipient "parents", of offspring and of those who participate in the process of reproduction through new technologies.

The Board urges that such a uniform or model law be drafted by the National Conference of Commissioners on Uniform State Laws, the American Law Institute, or some other qualified body. Because of the complex nature of the subject matter, however, the Board is aware that the task may be a major undertaking and suggests that the Department consider providing funds for drafting the legislation. Since the purpose is to safeguard the health and welfare of children and their families, it appears to be an appropriate project for Departmental support.

[FR Doc. 79-18925 Filed 6-15-79; 8:45 am]
BILLING CODE 4110-12-M

Index